What Experts are Saying...

"*Eat Right When Time Is Tight* is a must-have for time-starved women everywhere who want to eat well, stay focused and energized, and achieve and maintain a slimmer physique. Patricia has put together a smart, enjoyable read that's jam packed with practical, real-world, science-based nutrition and lifestyle tips women can easily fit into their harried lives wherever, whenever they eat. I highly recommend it!"

--ELISA ZIED, MS, RD, CDN, past Spokesperson for the American Dietetic Association and author of *Nutrition At Your Fingertips, Feed Your Family Right!,* and *So What Can I Eat?*

. . . .

"A wealth of common sense solutions. Patricia Bannan serves up nuggets of nutrition that a busy woman needs to succeed."

--LORI CORBIN, nutrition reporter, KABC-TV Los Angeles

. . . .

"This book is not a fad. It's a plan you'll want to stick with for the rest of your (busy) life."

--JEANNE GOLDBERG, PhD, RD, professor and director of the Graduate Program in Nutrition Communication, Tufts University

. . . .

"A timely tome for women everywhere who are overworked, overscheduled, and over trying any more fad diets. This book is packed with easy, proven, smart strategies that will get you slim and healthy in no time at all!"

--KATE GEAGAN, MS, RD, America's green nutritionist and author of *Go Green, Get Lean*

. . . .

"Patricia Bannan's simple strategies and solutions will save you time, boost your energy, improve your mood, and better your short-term and long-term health."

--DR. STEVE SALVATORE, medical correspondent/anchor, PIX Morning News New York

"If you have little time for cooking, it's nice to know there's a guide that can help. Patricia Bannan's meal ideas and strategies are clever, satisfying, and naturally nutritious."

--JACKIE NEWGENT, RD, CDN, culinary nutritionist and author of *The All-Natural Diabetes Cookbook* and *Big Green Cookbook*

....

"*Eat Right When Time Is Tight* uncovers the Holy Grail of weight loss on the go: A complete, yet simple plan that will actually work for you — and will keep on working. Patricia has created a very doable regimen that shows you how to achieve a healthy mindset, healthy body, and healthy relationship with food, regardless of how much time you have to spend."

--ANNE M. RUSSELL, Editor-in-Chief, VIV magazine

....

"Dietitians know that the strongest predictor of weight loss success is personal motivation. Patricia's brilliant strategies will keep you really motivated to lose weight the healthy way."

--CAROLYN O'NEIL, MS, RD, former CNN Food & Health correspondent, registered dietitian and co-author of: *The Dish on Eating Healthy and Being Fabulous!*

....

"In this book, Patricia helps busy readers conquer the time barrier for good. Her tips and tricks make it easy to eat natural, whole foods on-the-go."

--CYNTHIA SASS, MPH, MA, RD, CSSD, registered dietitian and New York Times bestselling author

....

"*Eat Right When Time Is Tight* is the perfect book for any time-pressed woman striving for optimum health and a slimmer physique. I love that it's full of practical and realistic nutrition tips based on science. As a busy Mom this makes my life a whole lot easier to keep on track and be the best that I can be. I highly recommend it!"

--TRACEY MALLETT, fitness expert and author of *Super Fit Mama and Sexy in 6*

"The meals and strategies are healthy and realistic, and now right at my fingertips. I expected nothing short of a fantastic guide to healthy living on the go from Patricia. And here it is: a fun, entertaining, and easy to use book based on the latest scientific information. Thank you, Patricia!"

--LINDA CIAMPA, RN, freelance correspondent
and producer for CNN Private Networks

....

"Every trainer knows working out is only part of the equation. Patricia Bannan's tips and tools will keep you fit inside and out, both physically and nutritionally."

--KATHY KAEHLER, celebrity fitness trainer,
author and creator of Sunday Set-Up™

....

"At last, a guilt-free book packed with good nutrition and weight loss secrets and tips for the time crunched person. Patricia Bannan has compiled a treasure trove of wonderful suggestions of healthy foods that go the distance whether you are on the go, on the road, trying to lose weight or just need a quick meal at home."

--KATHLEEN ZELMAN, MPH, RD, LD,
award-winning nutrition journalist

EAT RIGHT
WHEN
TIME IS TIGHT

150 Slim-Down Strategies and No-Cook Food Fixes

PATRICIA BANNAN, MS, RD

EAT RIGHT
WHEN
TIME IS TIGHT

150 Slim-Down Strategies and No-Cook Food Fixes

PATRICIA BANNAN, MS, RD

Printed in the United States of America
ISBN: 978-1-935254-29-4

Cover and Book Design by Tara Long
First printing, 2010

Dedication

To my parents Joanne and Bill, for their unwavering support and unconditional love.

Acknowledgements

Every book represents the work of not only its author, but dozens of others who play pivotal roles behind the scenes. I'm grateful to so many people who helped make this book a reality:

First, thank you to Kelly James-Enger, for effortlessly and patiently using her brilliance to bring my book to life. This book would not have happened without her and I am forever grateful.

Thank you to my publishers Dee and Sammie Justesen, for doing everything in their power to make this book a success; and to Nadene Carter for lovingly putting the words into print.

Thank you to my literary agent Krista Goering, for representing me and for finding such a lovely home for this book.

Thanks also to the fantastically talented and dedicated Tara Long, for her beautiful book design – both inside and out.

Thank you to my spokesperson agent, Beth Shepard, for help with the concept for the book and for years of creative ideas and support; and my publicist Mary Lengle, for opening doors, booking interviews, and being my sounding board every step of the way.

Thanks also to Jackie Newgent, for her culinary expertise and brainstorms; Jill Brown, for putting the fire into me to write a book and coming up with the catchy title; Caroline Gottesman, for her creativity in helping develop the meal plans; Susan Dopart, for her expert edits on the meal plans and professional mentoring;

and Kate Geagan, Nancy Tringali Piho, and Ellie Krieger, for their generous referrals.

A special thank-you to all who shared real-life experiences and strategies; your stories enriched these pages.

Another special thank-you to those who endorsed the book and inspire and motivate me to be a better communicator: Linda Ciampa, Lori Corbin, Kate Geagan, Jeanne Goldberg, Kathy Kaehler, Tracey Mallett, Jackie Newgent, Caroline O'Neil, Anne M. Russell, Dr. Steve Salvatore, Cynthia Sass, Kathleen Zelman, and Elisa Zied.

And finally, I acknowledge my family: my parents, Bill and Joanne; and Glenn, Maia, and Casner. Thank *you* for a lifetime of laughter, love, and support.

Table of Contents

EAT RIGHT?

Who Has Time?

You'd eat healthier, if only you had the time. A quick glance at your Blackberry tells you that will happen sometime between today and—exactly never.

You're not alone. Today's women have the same twenty-four-hour days their moms and grandmothers did, but our to-do lists are much longer—and always growing. Women are overbooked, overloaded, and overwhelmed, so it's no surprise that eating well is a challenge. And let's not forget the guys. They face longer hours at work, more family pressures (whether they're parents or not), and a host of issues (think mortgage meltdowns, keeping up with technology, and an ever-changing, insecure work landscape) their dads didn't have to worry about.

Ask today's woman about her day and you'll hear "Busy." "Crazy." "Insane!" Sure, you may *want* to eat better, lose weight, or set a better example for your kids, but these noble goals fall by the wayside when you're dealing with an iPhone that chirps every two minutes.

If this is ringing a bell (or lots of them), take heart. I'm here to help. You *can* eat better, no matter how busy you are, how many projects are pending at the office, and how many kids tug at your sleeves. My simple strategies and solutions will save you time, boost your energy, improve your mood, and better your short-term and long-term health. You'll even shed pounds in the process — without suffering.

Weight loss without suffering? More energy? Better health? Happier outlook? You think this sounds too good to be true? Well, it isn't — and this plan comes with a hidden bonus. These strategies not only *save* time — in the long run they *give* you time. By adopting these strategies you'll gain time and improved productivity in the short run and, thanks to improved health, you will add more time and better quality of life in the long run.

I want you to know I've struggled with many of the issues you face. I'm not a naturally skinny dietitian, model, or actress blessed with great genes telling people how to eat right while I nosh on whatever I want. I grew up a chubby, freckled-faced kid (although not so chubby by today's standards — kids are heavier than ever before). I started dieting my freshman year of high school and lost weight. I got attention for it and felt good. To keep the weight off I had to cut even more calories, but I stopped losing weight. This wasn't something I could maintain, so I ended up gaining back all the weight.

By the time I reached my twenties, I vowed to find a healthy way to lose weight and keep it off. That's why I decided to study nutrition in college and later become a registered dietitian. I wanted to absorb everything I could learn about the science and psychology of eating right. Now I'm passionate about helping people eat better and reap the rewards, including weight loss, better mood, more energy, improved health, and higher self-esteem.

Embracing these strategies provided an unexpected payoff: more time, plus the energy to make the most of that time. Today, in my late 30s, I don't have to learn about nutrition. I know what and how to eat and how to make the most of my minutes, nutrition-wise. And this has paid off in a variety of ways. I'm fit and healthy but I'm not a "twig" and never will be. Sure, I have to work to stay healthy and fit, which means making smart choices (at least most of the time) and exercising even when I don't feel like it. And while I have "fat days" like everyone else, I know how to get back on track—even when I'm working fourteen-hour days or constantly on the road.

You can learn how to do the same thing. Once you start embracing the Master Strategies, mini-strategies, and meal suggestions in the following chapters, you'll develop healthier eating habits that stay with you for good. While you'll invest time in reading this book and putting the strategies into place, once they become habits you'll boost your own personal Time Factor and discover you have more time in your day and you're more productive overall.

The Ever-Shrinking Day: Your Biggest Eating Obstacle

66My biggest obstacles to eating right and keeping the weight off are two-fold: time and my husband. After a twelve-hour day door-to-door, the last thing I want to do is make a meal. That means I either grab fast food on the way home or put the hubby in charge of dinner. The former means I might choose something "healthy" like a soup or salad from Panera, which can still total 1,000 calories, and the latter means a heaping portion of meat, usually red, alongside a giant potato (note a general lack of any veggie—or anything of the green, leafy variety).99

—Jill, 28, corporate communications writer

Ever felt like being overweight isn't your fault? You're actually not far off. If you're a typical woman, you face five major hurdles that make it more difficult (or nearly impossible) to eat more healthfully. (Most men, on the other hand, struggle with four obstacles—they don't worry about dieting as women do.) Lack of time is by far the biggest issue for both women and men. This is what I call The Ever-Shrinking Day.

If you run out of time and energy long before you run out of things to do, you're in good company. According to stress expert Alice C. Domar, Ph.D., the average woman worries about twelve things in a typical day while men worry about three. From the moment you roll out of bed in the morning, you're racing to get things done whether you're trying to make it to work on time or get the kids ready for school (and then get to work on time), or simply manage your busy household. When you consider that list of priorities, eating well or even eating better may slip to the bottom. You probably feel guilty, which adds yet another worry to your list.

The number one excuse (I mean reason) for not exercising is "lack of time," followed closely by "lack of energy." Lack of time is also the top reason for not eating better. According to a recent survey by the American Dietetic Association, only 43 percent of people believe a healthy diet and regular exercise are important *and* are doing all they can to consume a healthy diet. Another 38 percent feel maintaining a healthy diet and regular exercise is important, but they haven't taken "significant action" to eat a healthy diet. In other words, they're thinking about an improved diet, but aren't doing much about it.

The second reason people don't eat as well as they'd like? They say they need more *practical* tips to help them eat right. (Stay tuned ... you're going to find dozens of practical tips in the chapters that follow.)

I wasn't surprised by the second finding, because I see people struggle with this every day. We're inundated with nutrition information, but how do we know what to believe? Chocolate is bad for you, right? No, wait—it's actually loaded with antioxidants. Carbs are the enemy ... no, carbs are fine as long as they're the "right" kind of carbs. Swear off meat in favor of fish ... wait, some of that fish is loaded with poisonous mercury. It's hard enough for dietitians to keep up with the science, and that's our full-time job.

And honestly, who has time to overhaul a diet? No one I know has a spare weekend (let alone a week or more) to spend learning how to cram good nutrition into a busy lifestyle, even with the promise of more time at the end. So, if you're busy and overloaded, you simply shove your concerns to the back burner and promise yourself *one day* you will eat better. (And one day, you'll write that novel ... and redo your kitchen ... and start exercising regularly ... and learn to mediate, right?) If that's you, hello "one day," because you're reading the right book. We're in this together and we're going to get you out of your "fat pants" and into your skinny jeans for good.

THE FEARSOME FOUR: THE OTHER FAT FACTORS

If only lack of time kept you overweight, tired, and unhealthy, that would be one thing. But for most people, four other factors play a major role in your weight, food intake, and energy level. Those Four Fat Factors are:

- The Evil Environment;
- The Stress Factor;
- The Sleepless Night; and
- The Diet Drive. (If you're a guy, chances are you don't have to worry about this one.)

The Evil Environment

66 My main problem is the junk food available at work. My weight goes up and down in direct correlation to how well-stocked our snack bar is. I need to take time to pack a healthy lunch and avoid the temptations to eat junk food when I find myself hungry during my workday. 99

—*Stephie, 39, police officer*

Never before have you had so many choices and been so surrounded by food. It's difficult to eat healthy. Research proves that the more food we see, the more we eat—and food is literally everywhere. (When the checkout aisles at Best Buy are stocked with candy bars and bags of licorice, something is off.) So it's no surprise to learn we're eating more than ever before. According to the U.S. Department of Agriculture (USDA), Americans now consume an average of 523 more calories per day than in 1970. In 1970, the average person ate 2,234 calories a day. By 2007, most of us were scarfing down 2,704 calories a day, without realizing it.

Where do we get these extra calories? We're simply eating more food. Studies show we tend to eat what's put in front of us (didn't your mom always tell you to clean your plate?), and most of us underestimate how many calories we consume. And portion sizes just keep growing, both in restaurants and at home. A study in 2003 found that a typical restaurant cookie was 700 percent larger than the suggested USDA portion size. That is one big cookie. But if you actually eyeballed that cookie, you'd probably think it was maybe the size of two "normal" cookies, not seven.

This "portion distortion" affects us when we eat at home too, because plates, bowls, and even juice glasses are bigger than ever before. When you automatically pour a bowl of cereal, chances are you're eating more than one serving, but that fact never crosses your mind. Head to work and you face a minefield of tempting treats: doughnuts, pastries, and sweets in the break room, vending machines loaded with salty and sweet treats, catered-in boxed lunches, and the ever-popular celebrations (with cake, of course).

If you travel, you deal with the stress of being on the road and limited options, not to mention jet lag, delayed flights, and traffic hassles. Even if you're a stay-at-home mom or run a business from your house, the kitchen beckons. Every mom will testify to the ubiquitous nature of the kiddie snack food (i.e. Goldfish crackers, fruit roll-ups, and juice boxes) you can't leave home without.

Those are the biggest environmental factors, but we also face less obvious ones. For example, what do large plates, dimly lit rooms, fast music, and television have in common? They all make you eat more. Sharing a meal makes you eat about 44 percent more than if you dined alone—and the more people you eat with, the more food you consume. Don't feel discouraged or think you're doomed to a life of eating alone under bright lights in a sterile, silent room. One of my Master Strategies addresses how to safeguard your environment, and you'll learn how to make eating right easier. In the long run you'll save time because you'll safeguard your environment out of habit.

The Stress Factor

66 I actually do not eat at all when I'm stressed. When something stressful is happening around me, I won't eat until I feel more settled, and by then I've gone hours or sometimes a whole day without eating something. After that, I overeat and go for carbs. 99

—Katie, 36, teacher

Today you're likely to feel more stressed than ever before. A recent American Psychology Association poll found more people reporting physical and emotional symptoms of stress than during the previous year—and nearly fifty percent said their daily stress levels increased. Even people who don't actually feel stressed are likely to experience stress-related physical symptoms such as fatigue, irritability, anxiety, headaches, depression, and lack of interest.

The first part of the problem: we're chronically stressed. The second part is what we do when we're stressed. Four in ten women and three in ten men turn to food for comfort, and research suggests chronic life stress is associated with preferring calorie-rich and nutrient-poor foods that are high in fat and sugar. If you've ever munched away your troubles with a bag of chips and salsa or dove headfirst into a plate of chocolate chip cookies after a fight with your husband, you know this already. Guys may turn to a burger and fries, but the desire to distract yourself with food is the same.

Chronic stress may also increase your risk of weight gain, which then creates more stress because you're worried about being fat. Even minor daily hassles like misplacing your cell phone or having an argument with a co-worker can drive you to the cookie jar or vending machine. And if you're attempting to lose weight, you're even more likely to snack in reaction to stress. Researchers tell us stress increases the production of the hormone cortisol, which research shows increases your body's likelihood of storing abdominal fat, or belly fat, the place it's most detrimental to your health.

All that stress makes you more likely to reach for junk and less likely to stick with well-intended eating habits. You probably already know stress impacts your productivity, which means you're not making the most of your limited hours when you spend a day putting out fires at work or dealing with preschooler meltdowns. In short, the better you manage your stress, the better you'll feel— and the more you'll get done.

The Sleepless Night

66 Even as a baby, my son was never a good sleeper. Now, at 4 years old, he still wakes up during the night several times a week. He does go back to sleep, but I often lie awake for several hours ... and fall asleep just before I have to get up. The next morning, I'm exhausted and starving, and wind up snacking throughout the day to give myself energy. At least that's what I tell myself. 99

—*Kelly, 43, business owner*

Another often-overlooked obstacle to eating better has nothing to do with your diet but everything to do with your overall health and mood. It's called sleep. Get enough, and your immune system and metabolism function effectively. Yet most people skimp on sleep, either because they're busy or because they don't sleep well.

While recent stats tell us that two-thirds of people experience sleep problems at least a few nights a week, women are more prone to sleep disorders than men. Four in ten experience sleep problems every night, or almost every night. Nearly fifty percent of women wake up feeling "unrefreshed" at least a few nights a week, and three in ten either wake up and can't fall asleep or have difficulty falling asleep at least a few nights a week.

When it comes to total number of ZZZs, you probably don't get enough. Sleep needs vary, but according to the National Sleep Foundation, four in ten Americans get less than seven hours a night. Twenty percent of men and twenty-six percent of women say they're not getting the sleep they need to function at their best, and more than half say they get a good night's sleep less than half the time.

This lack of quality sleep actually makes you more likely to gain weight and take in excess calories during the day. According to one long-term study, the fewer hours a night a woman slept, the more likely she was to become obese. A review study that looked at 36 studies on sleep and weight gain found short sleep duration was independently linked to weight gain. Lack of sleep impacts your weight in the short-term as well. Another recent study found that restricting sleep even for a few nights makes you hungrier, more likely to have food cravings, and increases your caloric consumption—the perfect recipe for weight gain. And that doesn't take into account the impact lack of sleep has on your mood, memory, and attention span. In short, the fewer minutes you spend asleep, the more likely you are to feel hungrier and make poor food choices the next day.

This isn't just a matter of poor choices. A sleep-deprived brain doesn't function optimally, so you don't think as well and your productivity takes a nosedive. Deliberately sacrificing an hour or two of sleep may actually be counterproductive, as you wind up getting less done during those "extra" hours of being awake. Taking the time to get quality sleep isn't a waste of your time: rather, it gives you more time by making your non-sleeping hours more productive. And you'll have more years to be more productive, since sleep increases your longevity.

The Diet Drive

❝I've been all across the board as far as diets go. I'll be disciplined for a couple of weeks at a time, and then I'll binge.❞

—*Julie, 34, stay-at-home mom*

If you wish you could wake up one morning and magically find yourself 10 (or 20) pounds lighter, you have a lot of company. Our bodies (or more accurately, what's wrong with them) are constantly on our minds, and for most women that means wanting to lose weight. A recent survey of more than 3,000 women found 84 percent of women *believe* they're overweight. (In reality, 65 percent of women are actually overweight or obese.) A mere 13 percent say they're at their ideal weight. And these women are more concerned about their diet and body weight than anything else. While more than half were concerned about their diet and weight, less than a quarter worried about cancer or heart disease.

Self magazine conducted a study of 4,000 women between the ages of 25 and 45. They found 75 percent of women had an unhealthy relationship with food, their bodies, or both. Many of these women were actually at a healthy weight, but two-thirds of them were trying to lose weight regardless. Four in ten skipped meals to try to lose weight, and the same number admitted that worrying about what they eat and their weight interfered with their happiness.

I'm talking about women for a reason. Body dissatisfaction is much more a "woman thing" than a guy thing. While most men wouldn't mind dropping a few pounds, it's usually low on their radar. The typical guy doesn't obsess over his pants size or start a new diet every Monday.

And that's an advantage, actually, because diets don't work. Not in the long term, anyway. While you may lose a few pounds, unless you change your eating habits for good, you're likely to regain any lost weight once you return to eating "normally." Yet it's so easy to fall for the latest "breakthrough" plan. You have the "Oh, my God" moment when your favorite jeans don't fit, or you try on a swimsuit, or get weighed at your annual checkup. You launch an all-out weight loss regime, usually based on the latest strategy you've read about or seen on TV. And it works ... for a little while, anyway.

Problem is, these restrictive diet plans are often difficult to follow in the short-term, let alone long-term, and after a week or two you're hungry, tired, cranky, and sick of the food you're eating. After one particularly stressful day, you "blow it" and eat your way through the pantry, only to feel lousy the next day. (Researchers actually have a name for this—it's called the "what the hell" effect. As in, you slip off your diet with a candy bar, then think "what the hell" and continue overeating with wild abandon.)

Then you start the diet again, opt for another "proven" plan, or decide to forget about weight loss for awhile. But you still feel discouraged about your weight, and disappointed (or even disgusted) with yourself. That's no way to eat—and no way to live.

And dieting adds a tremendous "time suck" to your already-overloaded day. When you're cutting calories or trying to follow the latest "plan," your weight is on your mind (or in the back of your mind) all day long. You're thinking about what you're eating, what you're not supposed to be eating (but wish you were), what you're going to eat next, when you're going to eat next. Think of how much time you waste trying to summon your emotional reserves and willpower to stick to a diet—and how much of your mental energy is spent on that task rather than everything else you need to do. If you can derail your own "diet drive," you'll not only be happier, but more productive in the long run. I guarantee it.

YOUR JAM-PACKED, OVERWHELMING, INSANE, WONDERFUL LIFE

Just as no two people think the exact same way, no two of us face identical eating challenges. Getting a handle on obstacles *you* face will give you a better idea of what's keeping you from eating better and which areas to focus on. Take this quick quiz to help determine your personal eating minefields:

1. *I eat breakfast:*
   ____a. Every morning.
   ____b. Most mornings.
   ____c. If I have time.
   ____d. Rarely, if ever.

2. *I travel:*
   ____a. Never.
   ____b. Rarely.
   ____c. Frequently.
   ____d. At least once a week—I spend half my life on the road.

3. *I'm on a diet to lose weight:*
   ____a. Never—but I do try to eat healthfully.
   ____b. Occasionally.
   ____c. Often—let's just say I start one every Monday.
   ____d. About 100 percent of the time—I live on a diet.

4. *I eat in the car:*
   ____a. Rarely.
   ____b. Once in a while.
   ____c. Often.
   ____d. My car? You mean my kitchen on wheels? In other words, constantly.

5. *On a typical day, I feel:*
   ____a. Alert in the morning, with an energy dip in mid-afternoon.
   ____b. Alert in the morning, but become tired as the day drags on.
   ____c. Tired when I wake, though after a cup of coffee or a dose of caffeine I feel better—for a little while.
   ____d. Tired all day—I never seem to get enough rest.

6. *In the past month, I've had trouble sleeping:*
   _____a. Rarely.
   _____b. Occasionally.
   _____c. At least once a week.
   _____d. Several times a week—it's a real problem.

7. *How often do you eat out (including fast food)?*
   _____a. Rarely.
   _____b. Several times a week.
   _____c. At least once a day.
   _____d. More than once a day.

8. *At work, you:*
   _____a. Have a stash of healthy snacks in your desk.
   _____b. Try to bring a healthy lunch occasionally.
   _____c. Try to avoid the vending machines ... and usually succeed.
   _____d. Find yourself gravitating toward the break room (Doughnuts! Cookies! Leftover birthday cake!) on a regular basis.

9. *How often do you count calories or restrict certain kinds of foods (like carbohydrates)?*
   _____a. Never—I try to eat healthfully and don't worry about calories and fat.
   _____b. When I'm trying to lose weight, which occurs several times a year.
   _____c. Almost every day—unless it's the weekend.
   _____d. Every day—I'm always worried about what I'm eating.

10. *How often do you sit down and take twenty minutes or more to enjoy a meal?*
    _____a. At least once a day.
    _____b. Almost every day.
    _____c. Several times a week.
    _____d. Almost never—I don't have that kind of time.

11. *How do your body weight and mood correlate?*
    _____a. Neither seems to impact the other.
    _____b. When unhappy, I lose weight—I have no appetite.
    _____c. When I'm happy, I tend to lose weight without trying.
    _____d. When I'm unhappy, I can tell—I turn to food for comfort and put on weight.

12. **It's 3:30 p.m. and you're starving, though you had a big lunch. You:**
   ____a. Have a healthy snack, such as a piece of fruit and a string cheese.
   ____b. Grab what appears to be the least fattening option from the vending machine—a bag of mini-pretzels.
   ____c. Check out the break room or your fridge for something sweet—you need a quick sugar rush.
   ____d. Distract yourself—after that lunch, you refuse to eat again until dinner.

13. **It's a rainy Saturday and you have a few hours to yourself. You:**
   ____a. Pull out the book you've been meaning to read for ages.
   ____b. Grab a cup of coffee and a magazine.
   ____c. Read a few pages of your magazine, and fall asleep.
   ____d. Pass out before page 5.

14. **How often do you exercise?**
   ____a. Several times a week or more.
   ____b. Two or 3 times a week.
   ____c. Once a week.
   ____d. Does taking this quiz count as exercise? In other words ... never.

15. **How would you describe your stress level?**
   ____a. Manageable most of the time.
   ____b. Depends on the day.
   ____c. Pretty high.
   ____d. Um ... 12 on a scale of 1 to 10.

Give yourself 1 point for each A answer, 2 points for each B answer, 3 points for each C answer, and 4 points for each D answer. If you scored 15-20, you're facing fewer challenges than the average person; if you scored 21-30 points, you handle eating challenges fairly well, but could improve some of your habits; if you scored 31 to 42 points, you're facing a lot of challenges to eating more healthfully; and if you scored more than 43 points, you face challenges on all sides. For a closer look at your personal challenges, look at your answers to these questions. The more points you score for each obstacle, the more of an issue it may be for you.

Questions 1, 4, and 10 address *The Ever-Shrinking Day*.

Questions 2, 7 and 8 address *The Evil Environment*.

Questions 11, 14, and 15 address *The Stress Factor*.

Questions 5, 6, and 13 address *The Sleepless Night*.

Questions 3, 9, and 12 address *The Diet Drive*.

WHAT'S NEXT?

Now you have a better idea of why eating healthfully is such a challenge—not just for you but for nearly every person your age. Fortunately eating better doesn't mean overhauling your entire diet or paying attention to every morsel—I know you don't have time for that. In the next chapter, you'll learn about ten Master Strategies that will help you improve your diet, increase your energy level, boost your mood and your productivity, and gain quality time in your life. Read on for how you can eat better—starting now.

PATRICIA BANNAN

TAKE 10:

The Master Strategies to Eat Right when Time is Tight

Forget rigid diet plans. Eating right when time is tight starts with a handful of proven, simple strategies that will improve your nutrient intake, energy level, ability to handle stress, and waistline, while giving you back precious minutes.

This isn't a "diet" plan per se—not if you think of a diet as something to go on, and eventually go off. Over time, following these strategies will result in weight loss and the reason isn't surprising. Eat more calories than your body can use and you gain weight. Eat fewer calories than your body expends (while not getting hungry or feeling deprived) and you lose weight. That's all there is to it.

How many calories should you consume? About as many as you'll use throughout the day. MyPyramid.com, USDA's site that provides proven, practical nutrition advice, gives the following calorie recommendations for men and women:

Males	Not Active	Active
age 19-30	2,400	2,600-3,000
age 31-50	2,200	2,400-3,000
age 51+	2,000	2,200-2,800

Females	Not Active	Active
age 19-30	2,000	2,000-2,400
age 31-50	1,800	2,000-2,200
age 51+	1,600	1,800-2,200

According to MyPyramid.com, "Not Active" means you get less than thirty minutes of moderate physical activity most days, while "Active" means you get thirty to sixty minutes of moderate activity most days. (Don't feel bad if you fall into the "Not Active" category. Most people do, but I'll help you jump into the Active group, I promise.)

In addition to the Master Strategies and mini-strategies, inside this book you'll find a variety of meal ideas and daily meal plans. No need to count calories with these strategies, but I'll give you the basic breakdown in case you're a habitual calorie-watcher.

I generally recommend three meals a day with two snacks. However, if your schedule is such that you choose to eat more or less often, that's fine—just stick with Master Strategy 8 and energize every three to five hours to maintain your blood sugar levels and avoid overeating at your next meal. The total calories of the meals are: breakfast, about 300 calories; lunch, about 400 calories; dinner, about 500 calories. The two snacks have 150-200 calories each, bringing your total daily intake to about 1500-1600 calories.

To lose a pound a week you need to cut calories by about 500 a day. You can do that by eating less, exercising more, or a combination of the two. For example, an active 37-year-old woman will maintain her weight by eating about 2,100 calories a day and will lose 1 pound a week eating 1,600 calories a day while maintaining the same activity level.

If you're a man, or an extremely active woman, or you find you're hungry all the time following my recommendations, double your breakfast meal (to about 600 calories) or add a snack or two each day. Following these meal plans or basing your days on similar meals will result in a slow, steady weight loss over time—and you won't have to waste time worrying about whether you should be following the latest get-thin-quick program.

We've been talking calories and weight loss, but now let's talk minutes and time. I'm about to introduce you to my Master Strategies in this chapter and, in further chapters, you'll learn about more than one hundred additional mini-strategies and meals. These ten general strategies embrace the basics of eating right when time is tight—and they will save you time in the long run as well, whether it's cutting the time you spend deciding what to eat, chasing down a meal, or worrying over your weight. As a result, the Master Strategies will boost your productivity and energy level throughout the day, giving you back time in the short run, and adding years to your life in the long run—healthy, productive years, giving you even more time to enjoy life.

When I work with clients one on one, I help them identify their biggest diet pitfalls, and then determine which of the Master Strategies will give them the biggest payoff. In other words, which will have the greatest impact on their diet, weight, and energy level. I often talk about the hidden Time Factor of nutrition as well. When you give your body the food it needs, provide energy all day long, and manage your stressful lifestyle, you not only save time—you actually gain it. That's the Time Factor.

So, let's take a look at my ten Master Strategies—and how you can determine whether adopting each one will make a significant difference in your weight, energy level, mood, and productivity. Checking your Time Factor for each Master Strategy will help you identify whether that strategy will not only improve your nutrient intake and energy level, but help you gain time back as well. You may already be using some of these Master Strategies without realizing it. If so, that's great news. But you'll also learn which ones will give the biggest return, time- and weight-wise.

MASTER STRATEGY 1:
COMBINE PROTEIN AND FIBER.

This is the first Master Strategy for an important reason: The typical woman eats far more carbohydrates than she needs, but skimps on fiber and may be short on protein as well. The typical guy gets plenty of protein but also comes up short on fiber. Yet the latter two are essential, not only for a healthy diet, but for sustained energy and satiety as well. When you include protein and fiber every time you eat, you'll feel fuller longer and maintain a more stable blood sugar level, which translates to less fatigue and fewer food cravings.

Picture "protein" and you probably think of meat. Yet other good sources of protein include dairy products, soy, beans, legumes, eggs, and nuts. In other words, you don't have to polish off a steak every night to get the protein you need—and it's easier to incorporate into your diet than you may realize. Any vegetarian can tell you that.

In addition to creating and maintaining muscle, protein helps create red blood cells and keeps your hair, skin, and fingernails healthy. It also helps produce antibodies to fight off bacteria, viruses, and germs, and helps keep your immune system running strong. Studies show that people low on protein are more likely to get sick than people who eat enough of this nutrient.

How much protein do you need? The U.S. Recommended Daily Intake (RDI) of protein for adult men and women is 0.8 gram per kilogram of bodyweight a day. A kilogram is 2.2 pounds, which means a 140-pound woman should aim for about 51 grams of protein a day, while a 190-pound man should aim for about 69 grams/day. If you work out regularly, you need more: In general, 1.2 to 1.4 grams of protein/kilogram of bodyweight, or about 76 to 89 grams of protein a day for a 140-pound woman, and 104 to 121 grams of protein a day for a 190-pound man.

Fiber is the other part of this Master Strategy. Health professionals recommend adults consume between 25 and 35 grams of fiber a day, but most people get less than half that amount— between 14 and 15 grams a day.

Fiber is essential for good health and plays an important role in weight loss and maintenance. Because they help fill your stomach and increase digestion time, fibrous foods make you feel fuller longer. Another bonus: fiber-rich foods like fruits, vegetables, beans, and whole-grains are loaded with vitamins and minerals, making them a healthy bet overall.

Fiber comes in two types—soluble and insoluble. Soluble fiber dissolves in water, becoming gummy, while insoluble fiber holds water. Soluble fiber acts like a sponge, helping mop up cholesterol, while insoluble fiber is more like an intestinal broom that helps keep you regular. Research suggests a high-fiber diet may decrease your risk of high cholesterol, high blood pressure, and some cancers— and simply consuming more fiber can help you lose weight, too. A review study looked at the research on adding fiber to a typical diet. Overall, published studies found that adding 14 grams of fiber to people's regular diets produced an average weight loss of more than 4 pounds in four months.

While manufacturers are now adding fiber to everything from ice cream, to artificial sweeteners, to water, your best fiber bets are foods that contain it naturally. Aim to eat at least five servings of fruits and vegetables each day. (See Master Strategy 5.) Sources of natural fiber include fruits, vegetables, beans, legumes, seeds, and whole-grains like oatmeal, barley, and rye.

Check your Time Factor:

(Total Time Factor possible: 10)

____*Give yourself 1 point* for each time you eat fiber during the day
(up to 5).

+ ____*Give yourself 1 point* for each time you eat protein during the day (up to 5).

= ____*What's your Time Factor?* If it's less than 6, this Master Strategy will definitely boost your Time Factor. Even if it's more than 6 but less than 10, you'll see a difference by adopting it. Already at 10? Great job!

Three easy ways to incorporate this Master Strategy:

- Include a fruit or vegetable (with some protein) at every meal and snack.
- Stash a whole-food bar in your bag for a quick snack to provide both fiber and protein. [See Sidebar, Get the Most Energy from Your Energy Bar, on page 107.]
- Go nuts! Nuts are naturally packed with both protein, fiber, and many other nutrients to keep you well-fueled and healthy. Limit your serving size to one ounce or one to two handfuls.

MASTER STRATEGY 2:
SAFEGUARD YOUR ENVIRONMENT.

Your very environment is out to get you—prodding you to eat when you're not hungry, nudging you to eat more than you want, and seducing you with high-fat, high-calorie foods. Safeguarding your environment means just that—making wherever you are more conducive to eating healthfully and less conducive to eating junk. Motivation is only one part of successfully managing your weight. You will have days when your motivation is low (or completely gone), and that's when this Master Strategy becomes imperative to your success.

When you have a toddler, you childproof your home. Here, you're going to fat-proof your home, office, and car. Of course you can't control every environment, but you can take steps to help yourself. For example, I tell clients to keep portion-controlled, 200-calorie snack packs of nuts and trail mix in their cars in case they're on the road and get hungry. I can't tell you how many times clients have told me this simple strategy has saved them from having to stop and order something less healthy—or getting so hungry they would go overboard at their next meal. Their "bag o' nuts" saves them time, too.

Another safeguarding strategy is based on the old standby, "out of sight, out of mind." In other words, don't keep fattening foods where you can see them. If you tend to inhale the bread basket at a sit-down restaurant, ask your waiter not to bring it—or take it away after you have one piece. Automatically split your dinner entrée into halves and save half for a doggy bag for tomorrow's lunch or dinner.

Remember that the more food that is put in front of you, the more likely you are to eat it—so make an effort to reduce your "food exposure" when you can.

Check your Time Factor:

(Total Time Factor possible: 10)

_____*Give yourself 5 points* if you always carry a healthy snack with you.

+ _____*Give yourself 1 point* for each time you change your food environment for the better during the day (i.e., stashing sweets and junk food out of sight, using smaller bowls or plates, asking for a half-portion when dining out) (up to 5).

= _____*What's your Time Factor?* If it's less than 5, this Master Strategy will significantly boost your Time Factor (and help you lose weight). A Time Factor of more than 5 can be improved, and if you're at 10, well done!

Three easy ways to implement this strategy include:

- Carry a "secret weapon," or a portable snack to keep on hand when you get hungry.
- Serve meals at home on smaller plates—you'll automatically eat less.
- Make your residence a "safe" environment by not bringing your biggest temptation, be it cookies or chips, home. If it's not there, you can't eat it.

MASTER STRATEGY 3:
MUNCH EVERY MORN.

I know you already know you *should* eat breakfast. But if you're too busy in the morning to prepare a meal or you're not hungry first thing, I'm going to let you off the hook—sort of. You don't have to eat "breakfast," per se. I just want you to eat every morning.

I think breakfast has a bad rap, especially among busy people. Who has time to whip up a couple of eggs, toast, milk and juice on a typical crazy morning? My clients certainly don't. And plenty of people just aren't hungry when they awaken. I understand that. All I want you to do is eat something that contains protein and fiber (Master Strategy 1) within two hours of waking up. That's it. That single simple step will boost your metabolism, improve your mood, and make you more likely to consume the calories your body needs (without going overboard) for the rest of the day.

If you're counting every calorie, you may think going without breakfast will help you lose weight. In fact, the opposite is true. Eating a healthy breakfast every morning will make you more likely to shed pounds and keep them off. Statistics from the National Weight Control Registry, which tracks the habits of people who lost more than 30 pounds and kept the weight off, reveal that 78 percent of successful "losers" eat breakfast every morning. A mere four percent never eat breakfast.

You *think* you're saving calories, but when you skip breakfast, you're more likely to eat impulsively and overeat later in the day, which is bad news for your waistline. Eating in the morning also helps you think more clearly. The reason is simple—your brain runs on glucose, or sugar. When you awaken, your blood sugar levels are low because you haven't eaten for eight to twelve hours. Studies show that eating breakfast positively affects tasks that require retaining new information. Breakfast eaters also tend to be less depressed and less emotionally distressed than people who don't eat breakfast. When your brain and body are properly fueled, you feel better emotionally and physically.

Eating breakfast also appears to help your immune system efficiently function. Forget the idea of a traditional breakfast and just get in the habit of munching every morn.

Check your Time Factor:

(Total Time Factor possible: 10)

_____*Give yourself 7 points* if you always eat breakfast.

+ _____*Give yourself 1 point* if you ate breakfast today.

+ _____*Give yourself 1 point* if your breakfast usually includes protein.

+ _____*Give yourself 1 point* if your breakfast usually includes fiber.

= _____*What's your Time Factor?* If it's less than 7, this Master Strategy will boost your Time Factor. If it's above that, you're on your way, and if it's a 10, excellent work—keep it up!

Three ways to implement this strategy:

- Carry a whole-food bar with you to eat at your desk. [See Sidebar, Get the Most Energy from Your Energy Bar, on page 107.]

- Keep instant oatmeal packets at work for a quick, healthy breakfast.

- Forget "breakfast" foods if they don't appeal to you. There's nothing wrong with a healthy sandwich or beans and brown rice in the morning if that sounds good to you.

MASTER STRATEGY 4:
EAT AWARE.

When you eat a meal while driving or working at your desk, you're ingesting calories, but can you say you are enjoying it? Not really. Eating on the go may be your default, but that's something you may choose to change—at least some of the time.

"Eat aware" has several meanings. First, make an effort to become more mindful when you eat—at least once a day. That means taking time to savor your food, even if it's just a turkey sandwich on rye. We multi-task to get more done, but when you eat and never pay attention to your food, you're more likely to feel unsatisfied after your meal, and more likely to eat again later searching for that satisfaction. Becoming mindful doesn't mean you have to assume a lotus position or savor the inner essence of every raisin you consume. I'm just asking you to spend an extra few minutes focusing on your food, its taste, how it smells, and the texture. You'll find you eat more slowly, enjoy your food more, and are satisfied with less. That's a good thing.

If you want to become more mindful of what you're eating, consider keeping a food journal. Research shows that simply writing down what you eat and when you eat it aids in weight loss efforts. It also makes you more likely to make healthy choices. Something about having to write down *"3:30 p.m., inhaled 6 Oreos"* helps keep you on the straight and narrow, nutrition-wise.

"Eat aware" also means being smarter about the food choices you make. Eat closer to the earth by choosing more whole-foods like fruit and vegetables and less food packaged in plastic (think chips, cookies, candy). Look for ways to support sustainable farms and buy locally-grown produce at the supermarket. You don't have to make every vegetable organic, but the more attention you pay to your food and how it's grown and treated, the healthier your diet will be in the long run.

I realize you don't have time to sit and savor every meal, or spend an hour at the grocery store comparing the labels on produce, and the last thing I want you to do is feel guilty about it. But making an effort to "eat aware" even once a day will help you start a new habit of eating more mindfully and making choices that are healthier for you—and our planet.

Check your Time Factor:

(Total Time Factor possible: 10)

____*Give yourself 2 points* for each time you ate and really focused on your food today (i.e., without reading, watching television, or working) (up to 6).

+ ____*Give yourself 2 points* if you ate something organic or locally grown today.

+ ____*Give yourself 2 points* if you took twenty minutes or more to eat a meal today.

= ____*What's your Time Factor?* If it's less than 6, this is a Master Strategy to adopt. Even if it seems like you're getting less done (because you're not multitasking while you eat), you'll enjoy your food more, feel more satisfied, and feel less stressed in the long run ... giving you more productive time. If it's an 8 or higher, good work!

Three ways to implement this strategy:

- Eat while sitting down (driving doesn't count) and doing nothing else (no TV, email, telephone, or reading) once a day.
- Buy organic and locally-grown foods when you can.
- Read the label on food products you buy often; aim for whole-foods containing simple ingredients that you understand.

MASTER STRATEGY 5:
VEG OUT AND FRUIT UP.

How many fruits and vegetables did you eat yesterday? And no, French fries don't count, even if the USDA says otherwise. If the number is less than the fingers on one hand, you need to eat more green (and yellow, and red, and orange, and purple).

While women tend to eat more produce than guys do, most still fall far short on the recommended amount for optimal health—which is at least five servings of fruit and vegetables a day. Sure, you probably already know fruits and veggies are loaded with vitamins, minerals, and antioxidants. But they're also loaded with fiber (Master Strategy 1), are the most nutritious source of carbs, and are super low in calories and fat.

Research proves people who eat diets high in fruits and vegetables are less likely to develop chronic conditions like heart disease, high blood pressure, and certain types of cancer. And, the more fruits and veggies you eat, the more likely you are to have a healthy body weight as well.

Part of this is likely due to the substitution theory—i.e., if you choose an apple for a snack, you're less likely to grab a bag of chips. Now, I get the fact that if you're craving chips, an apple isn't going to cut it ... but maybe dried apple crisps will. I realize fruits and vegetables aren't always easy to find, and veggies in particular can be a hard sell for many grown-ups.

If you've spent much of your life on a diet, you may associate vegetables with "diet food" and fruits with "high sugar" and resist incorporating them into your regular diet. Or maybe you just never liked veggies as a kid. Fruits do contain sugar, but they're also packed with nutrients for health and water, plus fiber that aids with weight loss. For my clients who are fruit-phobic or struggle with losing weight, I recommend limiting their fruit intake to two servings a day and loading up on as many veggies as possible.

Even if you've never been a vegetable fan, you can learn to like them—over time. Start by going with what you like. If you hate celery and cauliflower, don't eat them. Instead, choose veggies you enjoy and look for ways to make them more palatable (e.g., roasting, grilling, eating them in sandwiches, or with salsa or low-fat dip. Experiment with different vegetables—even if you don't like brussel sprouts, you may find you love fresh tomatoes and peppers.

Check your Time Factor:
(Total Time Factor possible: 10)

____*Give yourself 1 point* for every serving of fruit you ate today (up to 3).

+ ____*Give yourself 1 point* for every serving of vegetable you ate today (up to 5).

+ ____*Give yourself 2 points* if you ate at least 3 different colors of fruits and vegetables.

= ____*What's your Time Factor?* If it's less than 6, this is a Master Strategy to adopt. It may take time in the short run to make sure you consume more fruits and veggies, but the long-run time benefits make it worth the investment. And if your Time Factor is 8 (or higher!), keep it up! The more fruits and vegetables you eat, the better.

Three easy ways to incorporate this strategy:

- Carry portable fruit (boxes of raisins, dried banana chips, an apple) in your purse or briefcase.
- Opt for a vegetable-heavy dish (broth-based soup or a salad loaded with veggies) for lunch.
- Add vegetables (tomatoes, pickles, onions, sprouts) to sandwiches.

MASTER STRATEGY 6:
APPESIZE YOUR MEALS.

Think of a typical day: You're on the go from the moment you get up. You grabbed lunch on the run, but you can't even remember what you ate. Was it a veggie sandwich? A sub? A burger? Nothing? Finally, you sit down to eat dinner and before you know it, you've stuffed yourself. In less than ten minutes you inhale more calories than you've eaten all day.

That's where what I call an "AppeSizer" comes in. An AppeSizer is an appetite speed bump. And just as a cement speed bump slows your car, an edible speed bump slows your eating. An AppeSizer is something that's low in calories and takes time to eat. A bowl of broth-based soup, an apple, a handful of sliced veggies and spicy salsa—all make excellent AppeSizers.

Your stomach takes about twenty minutes to signal your brain it's had enough food. An AppeSizer starts that clock running and slackens your eating pace, helping you transition from the stresses and pressures of your day to enjoying your meal. In short, an AppeSizer curbs your appetite and lets you feel satisfied with less—without making an effort to control your consumption.

Check your Time Factor:
(Total Time Factor possible: 10)

____*Give yourself 3 points* if you took longer than twenty minutes to eat a meal (up to 9).

+ ____*Give yourself 1 point* if you consciously chose an AppeSizer-type food to take the edge off your appetite before a meal.

= ____*What's your Time Factor?* If it's less than 6, this is a Master Strategy to adopt. Again, it may seem to take time to use AppeSizers but the time you take will give you time back in the long run. If it's 7 or above, good work!

Three easy ways to incorporate this strategy:
- Have a bowl of broth-based soup before a meal.
- Order a cup of hot herbal tea while you're waiting for a meal; it will take time to drink and give you something to do instead of munching on bread or appetizers.
- Have a 100-calorie snack that includes protein before a big meal (e.g., 2-3 tablespoons hummus, 1 tablespoon nut butter, 1 cup nonfat yogurt, or 30 pistachios).

MASTER STRATEGY 7:
HYDRATE.

Coffee. Juice. Diet soda. Frappacino. You may be drinking all day long, but how much water are you actually consuming? Most Americans don't consume the amount their bodies need. Your body needs water to function normally (it's made up of 60 percent water by weight), and when you're dehydrated you may also feel tired, have trouble concentrating, or wind up eating more than usual, because your brain often misinterprets thirst as hunger.

Every cell of your body requires water. Water is also essential to convert food into energy, remove waste, regulate body temperature and hunger, and carry nutrients and oxygen throughout your body. Unfortunately, you can be dehydrated and not even realize it. By the time you actually feel thirsty, you're about two percent dehydrated. Dehydration is measured in percentages relating to body weight— for example, a 150-pound person who is 1 percent dehydrated has lost 1.5 pounds in water weight. It's easy to walk around chronically dehydrated without knowing it, and even mild dehydration can impact your day-to-day life. You may feel lightheaded, dizzy, tired, headachy, or have trouble focusing or concentrating. All are symptoms of slight dehydration.

So how much water should you be drinking? Probably more than you think, because an average sedentary person loses about 2.5 quarts of water a day through ordinary activity alone. And if you exercise, you lose between 0.8 and 1.5 quarts of fluid each hour as well. All this fluid should be replaced to maintain optimal hydration.

You've probably heard or read that people need eight 8-ounce glasses of water each day, but that's not necessarily true. You're better off checking your urine amount and color for a better read on your personal hydration status. Lots of light yellow urine means you're drinking enough. Scanty or dark-colored urine usually means you need more fluid. It can also mean you're taking vitamins you don't need, or a medication is throwing the color off.

One more thing—while water is always a good bet, you needn't rely only on H_2O to satisfy your fluid needs. Beverages like tea, soda, coffee, and juice all contribute to your daily total, as do foods like soup, fruits, and vegetables that are naturally high in water content. The benefit of water is that it has no calories, which is key for weight loss. But if you choose to hydrate with other beverages or foods, watch the added calories and sugar they contain. Drink more, and you may have to make more frequent bathroom stops, but it will be worthwhile in the way you feel.

Check your Time Factor:

(Total Time Factor possible: 10)

_____*Give yourself 1 point* for every glass of water, non-sugared tea, 100 percent juice, or low-sodium vegetable juice you drank yesterday (up to 10).

= _____*What's your Time Factor?* If it's less than 5, this is a Master Strategy to adopt. Staying hydrated with the right fluids will boost your energy level and productivity. Yes, you'll spend a little more time in the bathroom, but you'll gain time overall. If your Time Factor is 8 or above, good work.

Three easy ways to incorporate this strategy:
- Drink a big glass of water in the morning, after you brush your teeth.

- Keep a bottle of water in your bag, preferably in a stainless steel container.
- Keep tea bags at work and swap tea for coffee occasionally.

MASTER STRATEGY 8:
ENERGIZE IN 3-5.

This strategy is not only about *what* you eat but *when* you eat. The typical busy person eats little throughout the day and then overeats in the evening, but starving all day and binging at night is not only hard on your psyche, it's the most inefficient way to provide your body with the energy you need. Yet many of us follow this pattern of skimping throughout the day, only to overeat at night.

For optimal energy levels, you want to stay in "energy balance"— or close to it—throughout the day. That means providing your body with the amount of fuel it needs at regular intervals so you're neither overeating nor under-eating. Understanding how your body's blood sugar levels rise and fall explains why this is critical, whether you want to lose weight or simply have more energy and feel better throughout the day.

Normally if you eat something, your blood sugar, or glucose levels, will rise, level out, and then drop in about three hour units. If you don't eat every three hours or so, blood sugar begins to drop even further. Your *brain* knows you're stuck in a meeting and can't eat, but your *body* doesn't know that. It thinks you're in danger of starving. The more time that elapses before you eat, the lower your blood sugar falls. Then, when you do eat, you'll produce more insulin than normal because your cells are desperate for energy. Insulin works as the gatekeeper to help transport glucose into your cells, and the more insulin you make, the hungrier you feel—and the more likely you are to store extra calories as fat. That's the double-whammy of skipping meals. Not only do you feel crabby or tired from hunger, you're more likely to gain weight as a result.

When you stay close to energy balance, however, you keep your blood sugar levels relatively stable throughout the day, which means more consistent energy levels, less hunger, and a better mood. Instead of eating three meals a day, aim for three smaller meals and one or two snacks. Done right, snacking helps you maintain steady blood sugar levels and makes you less likely to overeat at your next meal.

If you're trying to lose weight, you might think the fewer calories a snack has, the better. But while a handful of carrot sticks may take the edge of your hunger for a few minutes, they won't keep you going for long. Snacks that include protein and fiber (Master Strategy 1) will give you sustained energy for hours.

Check your Time Factor:
(Total Time Factor possible: 10)

____*Give yourself 8 points* if you usually eat every three to five hours throughout the day.

+ ____*Give yourself 1 point* if you planned healthy snacks at the start of the day.

+ ____*Give yourself 1 point* if you had a healthy snack on you, or in your car, or at work—even if you didn't eat it!

= ____*What's your Time Factor?* If it's less than 8, this Master Strategy will boost your Time Factor. If it's 8 or above, keep it going!

Three easy ways to incorporate this strategy:
- Carry your secret weapon and "safeguard your environment" (Master Strategy 2) so you can sneak a snack if you need to.
- If it's been more than four hours, eat something healthy—even if you're not hungry yet. You'll keep your blood sugar from plummeting.
- Set a reminder on your phone or watch so you don't go more than five hours without eating.

MASTER STRATEGY 9:
SWEAT 30+.

This may seem counterintuitive, but one of the keys to eating better has nothing to do with the food you take into your body. It has to do with what you do with your body. Yes, I'm talking about exercise.

As I mentioned in Chapter 1, the number one reason for not eating better is lack of time, and such is the case with exercise as well. I don't know anyone who isn't aware that they *should* be exercising. Lack of knowledge isn't the problem—it's time and motivation. And if you can't find the time (or the drive) to work out, that's just one more thing to feel guilty about.

People who exercise regularly are healthier overall than those who don't. They're less likely to develop chronic diseases like heart disease, high blood pressure, high cholesterol, diabetes, osteoporosis, and many cancers. Yet thinking, "Yeah, yeah, I need to go sweat my butt off on the treadmill so I won't get diabetes twenty-five years from now" isn't that motivating.

Instead, think about the more immediate benefits of exercise. First off, it's a mood booster. People who work out are less depressed and less anxious than those who don't, and even short bouts of exercise improve mood and relieve stress. Although you can't work out once and lose 10 pounds (wouldn't that be great!), you can work out once and feel 10 pounds lighter emotionally.

Workouts also give you more energy long-term. If you launch an exercise program, yes, you'll feel tired after months (or years!) of riding the couch. But after about four to six weeks you'll notice a difference in your energy level. Activity makes your cardiovascular system more efficient, which means more oxygen gets to your brain and your muscles, and makes it easier to do everyday tasks like running to catch a flight or carrying six bags of groceries from the car.

Still not convinced? Then stop thinking of it as exercise—just think of it as becoming more active and moving more than you do now. Even walking more will help you sleep more soundly, maintain a healthy body weight, and encourage you to eat better as well. And let's not forget about vanity. Regular activity improves your looks and self-esteem. Exercise also boosts something called self-efficacy, or your belief in your own abilities. That's critical for *you* — the overloaded, overwhelmed, over-booked readers of this book. The more you have to do, the more faith you need in your ability to get things done.

Check your Time Factor:

(Total Time Factor possible: 10)

____*Give yourself 1 point* for each day you exercise for thirty minutes or more in an average week (up to 6).

\+ ____*Give yourself 2 points* if you worked out today.

\+ ____*Give yourself 2 points* if you made an effort today to be more active (e.g., taking the stairs when possible, taking walking/ stretching breaks at work, parking farther away).

= ____*What's your Time Factor?* If it's less than 6, this is a Master Strategy to adopt. Working out is a time-giver. Sure it takes time to do, but it gives you more time in the long run, boosting your Time Factor. If it's a 7 or more, keep up the good work!

Three easy ways to incorporate this strategy:

- Aim for ten minutes. Research shows that three ten-minute stints of activity provide the same health benefits as one continuous thiry-minute session.

- Wear a pedometer. See how many steps you're walking a day and gradually increase it by 500 each week until you reach 10,000 steps a day.

- Get an exercise buddy and hold each other accountable.

MASTER STRATEGY 10:
RECHARGE.

You know from chapter one (and from your own life) that you're under stress. Maybe not every single moment of every day—but you definitely experience stress on a regular basis. Stress can not only make you sick, it can make you fat as well.

Research shows stress contributes to high blood pressure and increases your risk of having a heart attack, stroke, or other disease—plus, it can add to your waistline.

Fat comes in two basic types: visceral fat, which is stored in the abdomen and pads your internal organs, and peripheral fat, which is stored just below the skin. While peripheral fat may not *look* attractive (it's responsible for those bulges on our hips and thighs), it's less risky to your health than visceral fat. Studies show people with more visceral fat, or belly fat, have an increased risk of developing heart disease, diabetes, high cholesterol, and other health issues.

Yet even women who tend to gain weight on their hips and thighs add fat around their middles when they're under stress. Why? When your body is stressed, you produce higher levels of stress hormones like cortisol and adrenaline. In turn, those hormones appear to increase the amount of visceral fat your body stores.

Stress impacts your body weight in less obvious ways, too. Picture this—you're driving to work and suddenly another car veers in front of you. You slam on the brakes and squeal to a stop, missing the car's bumper by inches. You gasp in fear and your heart pounds; a few minutes later, you feel shaky, weak, and nauseous. That's your body reacting to the perceived threat in what's called the fight-or-flight response, and it's likely to make you hungrier as a result.

As your cardiac, respiratory and central nervous systems all rev up, they require more fuel. While our ancestors may have needed those extra calories to fight off a saber-toothed tiger (or run away from it), the stressors of today usually don't require additional fuel to combat—and so those calories get stored as fat. The problem with chronic stress is that it provokes this kind of response continuously, and you wind up with a constant urge to eat.

Of course, stress-triggered eating binges have little to do with hunger or appetite. When you're stressed you lack the staying power to make smart food choices, and you may use food to distract yourself or make you feel better. That can mean eating starchy, sweet foods like cakes or fatty, salty foods like French fries. You're also likely to turn to comfort foods like potato chips, ice cream, cookies, and pizza when you're under pressure.

That's the bad news about stress and how you eat. The good news is, you can combat stress in a variety of ways, regardless of how busy you are. More on this in Chapter 8. With stress management, there is no one-size-fits-all approach—it's what works for *you*.

Check your Time Factor:

(Total Time Factor possible: 10)

____*Give yourself 2 points* if you took breaks throughout your day to manage your stress.

+ ____*Give yourself 2 points* if you laughed today.

+ ____*Give yourself 2 points* if you slept at least seven hours last night.

+ ____*Give yourself 2 points* if you felt calm or relaxed a good part of the day.

+ ____*Give yourself 2 points* if you used a stress-management technique (deep breathing, exercise, meditation, prayer) sometime today.

= ____*What's your Time Factor?* If it's 4 or less, this Master Strategy will definitely improve your Time Factor. Working toward a 10 will boost your Time Factor—and if it's a 10 already, stay Zen!

Three simple ways to implement this strategy include:

- Take two minutes to simply stop what you're doing and breathe. Inhale and completely fill your lungs so your belly swells. Then exhale completely. Even two minutes will slow your heart rate, breathing, and blood pressure, which creates a feeling of relaxation.
- Use laughter as medicine—the best medicine. Humor defuses stress and the stress hormones it produces. Surround yourself with light-hearted, funny people, watch a comedy, or "find the funny" in your daily life.
- Get a pet. Research shows pets calm us and lift our spirits.

YOUR MASTER STRATEGY WORKSHEET

Now that you've had a chance to learn more about the Master Strategies and your personal Time Factor for each, take a few moments to note which ones give you the most return on your time investment:

MASTER STRATEGY Current Time Factor (out of 10)

- Master Strategy 1: Combine protein and fiber._____
- Master Strategy 2: Safeguard your environment._____
- Master Strategy 3: Munch every morn._____
- Master Strategy 4: Eat aware._____
- Master Strategy 5: Veg out and fruit up._____
- Master Strategy 6: AppeSize your meals._____
- Master Strategy 7: Hydrate._____
- Master Strategy 8: Energize in 3-5._____
- Master Strategy 9: Sweat 30+._____
- Master Strategy 10: Recharge._____

Circle the ones you need to work on, and make a note of the date. Over time, you can revisit this sheet to check your progress. Stay aware of which Master Strategies will make the biggest difference in your weight, mood, health—and give you the most time back as well.

Identifying the Master Strategies that give you the biggest results will help you identify *your* priorities. Now that you know which ones to focus on, you'll learn dozens of specific ways to put them in practice so you'll eat better on the run, improve your Time Factor, lose weight, and feel fantastic in the process. From breakfast to dinner, from eating at home to eating on the road, from everyday meals to special occasions, you'll find practical, doable solutions for your busy life—and be able to eat right, regardless of how crazy your day is.

MORNING MUNCHIES:

The Breakfast Boost

"When I have time, I always try to cook breakfast and make it a sit-down meal. Taking the time to actually prepare something makes me feel more connected to my food and my health, and helps me make better nutrition choices later in the day. That sounds like something I stole from *Self* magazine, but it's true.

Lately, I've been on a big egg kick, so I'll normally have two scrambled eggs with a slice of wheat toast and a banana. I always try to include a protein, a carbohydrate (preferably a complex one), and a fruit (or if not that, then a small glass of juice). When I'm on the run, I pack a baggie of shredded wheat or some other high-fiber cereal, and a small serving of nuts. Even though meal bars are technically well-rounded in the nutritional sense, I try to avoid them—or at least the ones with loads of carbs and sugar. But, in a real pinch, I'm known to grab an energy bar."

—Alyssa, 23, freelance copy editor

Alyssa is one smart girl. Barely out of college, she's already figured out that not only is breakfast the most important meal, she mastered the art of fitting it into her day.

The Skinny on Breakfast Cereals

Cereal and milk is one of the most popular (and easiest) breakfasts out there. Whether you choose hot or cold cereal, this breakfast staple is an excellent opportunity to get whole grains, fiber, and vitamins and minerals into your body.

Only one problem: With the crowded, colorful, jam-packed cereal aisle, how do you possibly make sense out of those cereal options?

First, limit sugar. The less sugar your cereal contains, the better. Look for cereals with no more than 10 (5 or less is even better!) grams of sugar and at least 5 grams of fiber/serving. Check the ingredient list. You want to choose a cereal that contains a whole grain as the first ingredient. If you don't see the word "whole," the grains have been processed and are less nutritious.

Either cold or hot cereal can make a healthy breakfast, but the ones claiming to contain fruit may offer little actual fruit, with more fruit flavorings and artificial colors. Check the label, where fruit should be one of the first few ingredients. If it isn't, you're better off buying a plain cereal or oatmeal and adding your own fresh or dried fruit— you'll get less added sugar, more fiber, and more flavor (and nutrition) overall.

Finally, watch your portions, because it's easy to eat more cereal than you realize, especially if you use a large bowl. Measuring a serving a few times will help you eyeball the right portion size in the future. Some of my clients measure a serving size of their favorite cereal in their usual breakfast bowl, and then mark a line with a permanent marker so they know how to fill it each morning for time-saving portion control.

10 second take-away:

- Choose a whole grain cereal with the word "whole" listed as the first ingredient.
- Opt for cereals that contain 10 or fewer grams of sugar and at least 5 grams of fiber/serving.

THE BASICS OF BREAKFAST

Let's get down to the basics. Here you go:

Breakfast = good.

No breakfast = bad.

I'm joking ... sort of. Breakfast may be the meal most often skipped, yet from your body's point of view it's the most important. Consider this: your body has been fasting for at least eight hours or longer (unless you were prowling your kitchen for a 3:00 a.m. snack four hours before you got up). That means your stomach is empty and your blood sugar is low. Research shows that fasting enhances the subjective appeal of high-calorie foods over lower-calorie ones. That's why you crave carbs in the morning, and why people snatch up the cranberry scones, cinnamon rolls, and giant bagels at coffee shop counters. Carbohydrates are easily digested, making them a quick source of energy, but they lack the staying power of protein or fat.

So, your body craves carbs in the morning. Why not give it what it wants? I'm not saying to inhale an entire Entemann's coffee cake for breakfast, but plenty of different carbs will give you an immediate energy boost, plus nutrients to boot. The key is choosing high-fiber, whole-grain carbs (I'll tell you how to find them in a few pages) and tempering those carbs with some protein for steady, lasting energy. Later in this chapter, you'll find a list of quick, easy breakfasts on-the-run—and ways to make the best of less-than-healthy choices as well.

Consuming complex carbohydrates in the morning also increases the amount of a specific brain chemical, a neurotransmitter called serotonin. Serotonin causes a feeling of calm and relaxation, and carbohydrates increase the amount of serotonin your brain produces. So a breakfast that includes complex carbs not only provides immediate energy, but also helps give you a sense of calm, even on your most harried morning.

Boost Your Nutrient Intake

Your morning meal also presents an opportunity to improve your overall nutrient intake. Research shows people who don't eat breakfast have a much lower nutrient profile (meaning they take in smaller amounts of vitamins and minerals) than breakfast eaters. This is the easiest meal to eat healthy because it's the one you're most likely to control. Compare this to lunch and dinner, where you may be eating out or on someone else's schedule. Breakfast

Is Breakfast a Meal or a Snack?

Do you eat a "real" breakfast every day? Probably not. A recent survey found that more than half of people's breakfasts consist of one or two items. Only 38 percent of Americans said they viewed their breakfast as a full or complete meal, while 45 percent considered it a small or mini-meal. Another 5 percent of people considered it just a snack, while another 11 percent limited it to beverages such as coffee and fruit juice.

More than half of all breakfasts are consumed in less than ten minutes, so it's not surprising the vast majority of breakfast foods and beverages require no preparation or cooking. Here are the most popular breakfast foods and beverages consumed at home (and how likely they are to be consumed):

- Coffee -   32 percent
- Cold cereal - 32 percent
- Fruit juice - 26 percent
- Milk -   16 percent
- Bread -   15 percent

- Fruit -   13 percent
- Eggs -   12 percent
- Hot cereal - 9 percent
- Bacon -   4 percent
- Hot tea -   4 percent

The good news: all of the above foods are healthful if you choose wisely. As discussed earlier, go for high-fiber cereal, whole-grain bread, 100 percent fruit juice, and one percent or skim milk. Even bacon is okay on occasion if you choose a lean version like Canadian bacon.

gives you a great opportunity to "front-load" your day with healthy options like fruit, lean protein, and whole grains that are high in fiber and nutrients.

The Whole Truth about Whole Grains

Sure, you know you're supposed to eat whole grains, but that may be harder to do than you realize. While we eat plenty of grains, the typical American consumes less than one serving a day of whole grains—and whole grains provide a wealth of nutrients their refined versions lack. Plenty of research suggests a diet high in whole grains may help reduce your risk of developing heart disease and other conditions.

While all grains provide complex carbohydrates, vitamins, and minerals, whole grains offer more bang for your buck. The reason? A whole grain is actually a seed made up of three parts—the inner germ, from which a new plant would sprout; the endosperm, which makes up most of the grain; and the outside bran, containing most of the seed's fiber. Eating the entire grain means you get all the nutrients and all the fiber of the seed. Yet most grains are refined or processed, during which the endosperm and bran are eliminated. That means refined grains have fewer vitamins and minerals, and less fiber than whole grains.

Opting for whole-grain versions over their refined cousins is a simple way to improve your nutrient intake. But that's not always as simple as it sounds. Take the word "multi-grain." Sounds good, right? Well, it may mean that the product contains more than one grain but not necessarily whole grains. To be sure, check to see that the word "whole" is the first word listed in the ingredients.

Whole grains include barley, brown rice, wild rice, bulgur, oatmeal, whole wheat, and popcorn. Look for foods containing at least 3 grams of dietary fiber/serving, and aim for three 1-ounce servings every day.

10 second take-away:

- Look for the word "whole" to be listed first in the ingredients— anything else may not contain the entire grain.
- Aim for 3 servings of whole grains a day.

Nobody Ever Got Fat Eating Breakfast

Sure they did—if they ate the entire buffet table of sausage, pancakes, and gravy-soaked biscuits. But that's not what we're talking about here. Put your fears aside about gaining weight by eating breakfast. Sure, you'll put on pounds if you eat more calories than you expend. But you're more likely to burn off the calories you consume at breakfast than any other calories you take in throughout the day. And you're least likely to burn off the extra calories (i.e., more than your body requires) you consume at night, which is logical when you think about it. Contrast your busy day with your typical night spent in bed and you can see where you're expending most of your energy—unless your nightlife is way more exciting than mine.

Experts Agree ... Breakfast Makes you Smarter

Researchers have long studied the impact of breakfast on children's performance and attention span at school. Those results probably translate to grown-ups, and plenty of studies prove a strong correlation between eating breakfast and performing better at work.

- A study of nearly 400 middle school students found that regular breakfast eaters had higher grades, better memory, and higher levels of concentration than students who skipped breakfast.
- Another study, this time of high school students, found that students who ate breakfast were more alert and had higher levels of cognitive functioning than their peers who ate no breakfast.
- A study of more than 100 second-year medical students revealed that skipping breakfast (and skipping meals in general) was associated with fatigue.
- A study of college students in the United Kingdom found that students who consumed glucose drinks and watched a safety presentation recalled more than 20 percent more material than students who had a zero-calorie beverage instead.

Researchers aren't sure why breakfast has such an impact. In fact some studies show that skipping breakfast has no impact on certain

Lunching on Lunch Meat—Your Best Choices

A quick sandwich may be the most popular lunch around, and you can find dozens of different meats to put on your whole-grain bread. Look for meats that contain no more than 3 grams of total fat and no more than 1 gram of saturated fat per 2-ounce serving. Your best options are chicken, turkey, and roast beef.

Because processed luncheon meats are high in sodium and nitrates/nitrites (preservatives you should limit in your diet), check the labels and look for ones that contain no more than 500 mg of sodium per 2-ounce serving and no nitrates/nitrites. Certain brands contain no preservatives, so look for this claim on the label. If you can buy organic luncheon meat, even better—the organic standard means the meat contains no antibiotics or preservatives.

Another option is to grab a rotisserie chicken (which being recently cooked hasn't had preservatives added) and make sandwiches from it. And if you want to cut your salt content or need a vegetarian option, check out veggie versions of turkey, chicken, ham, and other meats. Vegetarian options are often made from soy, TVP (textured vegetable protein usually made from soy flour), beans, or a combination of non-meat proteins.

If you choose a vegetarian "meat" made from soy, look for those that contain whole soy instead of processed soy (i.e., "soy protein isolate"). Just as whole grains contain all the nutrients and fiber compared to refined or processed grains, "whole soy" retains all of the soybean's nutritional profile. And you can count "whole-soy-derived" lunchmeat toward the recommended 3 cups of beans and legumes you should eat every week.

10 second take-away:

- Choose lunch meats that contain less than 3 grams of total fat and 500 mg of sodium per 2-ounce serving.
- Whether you choose lunchmeat or lunch "meat," organic is your best bet as it will ensure you're getting zero preservatives or antibiotics in your sandwich meat.

aspects of thinking and reasoning. But we know eating breakfast raises your blood sugar levels, which appears to enhance short-term memory and may positively influence attention as well. Bottom line: When you break your fast, you supply your body and brain with energy and nutrients, and that can only be a good thing overall.

Beat Bitchiness with Breakfast

And here's another factor to consider. How often are you grumpy in the morning? Maybe it's not lack of sleep, a cranky toddler, or a rush project at work that's to blame … it's your empty stomach. Breakfast eaters are happier, less depressed, and less anxious than breakfast skippers. They also report better mood and feeling more sociable than those who survive on black coffee and adrenaline.

Fiber versus Fiber: What's the Difference?

How's your fiber intake? If you're like most people, you probably fall short. While dietitians recommend adults consume between 25 and 35 grams of fiber a day, most Americans get less than half that amount—more like 15 grams a day. Fiber is not only critical for good health and proper nutrition, it can play an important role in your weight loss arsenal as well.

What is fiber, anyway? It's the part of plant foods that cannot be digested, and falls into two categories—soluble and insoluble. The two types react differently in water. Soluble fiber dissolves in water and becomes gummy, acting like a sponge to soak up "bad" cholesterol. Insoluble fiber doesn't dissolve in water and acts more like a broom, essentially "sweeping" out your intestines and helping keep you regular.

A diet high in fiber may help reduce your risk of certain conditions like heart disease, high blood pressure, diverticulosis, and some forms of cancer. Fiber also helps with weight loss, because high-fiber foods make you feel full longer and take longer to digest.

Food manufacturers are responding to the growing desire for fiber by putting it in places you'd never think of—yogurt, juice, artificial

That's a side effect of that happy brain chemical, serotonin, working in their favor.

Eat Breakfast, Stay Healthy

Eating breakfast also helps keep your immune system functioning efficiently. At least one published study found breakfast eaters were less likely than breakfast skippers to catch a cold. Another study that surveyed more than 15,000 people found those who ate breakfast reported higher "health-quality of life" than breakfast skippers. They were healthier, and equally important, they felt healthier. The morning-munchers had better mental health than those who went without, and were less likely to become obese.

sweeteners, and even water. How is this possible? Because this new fiber is an "isolated fiber" like inulin or polydextrose. These purified fibers aren't the same as intact fiber found naturally in foods like fruits, vegetables, beans, and legumes. And while it may count toward the fiber content on the label, the jury's still out on the potential health benefits of isolated fiber. (Some studies suggest inulin may help boost the beneficial bacteria found in the digestive tract, but there's no evidence it promotes regularity or lowers cholesterol the way regular fiber does.)

The bottom line with fiber is that you're better off getting intact fiber from whole foods that naturally contain it, rather than from foods with fiber added as a marketing ploy. That means including fruits and vegetables, beans, legumes, whole grains, and nuts in your regular diet.

10 second take-away:

- Aim for at least 25 grams of fiber every day.
- Intact fiber (found naturally in high-fiber foods) is better overall than "isolated fiber" popping up in many processed foods.

Breakfast Makes You Skinny

I've saved the best news for last. As the above-mentioned study showed, eating breakfast actually makes it easier to lose weight—and maintain a healthy weight. A recent survey of 12,136 Americans revealed that people who ate breakfast actually consumed fewer calories over the course of a twenty-four-hour day than those who

Read All About It:
Understanding the Nutrition Facts Label

You know every packaged food is required to have a Nutrition Facts label, but do you know how to read that label, or what to look for? You don't need a degree in nutrition or chemistry to decipher these labels if you keep a few facts in mind.

First, check at the top of the Nutrition Facts label where it lists serving size, number of servings per package, number of calories, and nutrient information per serving. You may be surprised to find what you think is a serving (say a bag of chips) is actually two or three portions.

Checking the number of calories and fat grams will also help you determine how this food fits into your diet. You'll also find the amount of saturated fat, trans fat (although most manufacturers have removed trans fats from foods), and cholesterol the food contains (these are all things to limit) as well as nutrient information for certain vitamins and minerals.

The General Guide to Calories at the bottom of the Nutrition Facts label is based on a 2,000 calorie/day diet. The % Daily Value figures help you determine whether a serving of a food is high or low in that particular nutrient. According to the USDA, a food with more than 10 percent of the Daily Value of a nutrient is a "good source" of that nutrient and a food with more than 20 percent of the Daily Value of a nutrient is an "excellent source" of that nutrient. For example, one serving (or one cup) of milk provides 30 percent of your Daily Value for calcium, meaning milk is considered an excellent source of calcium.

Here's one more thing you should know about reading a food label: ingredients are listed in order of amount, so the higher up on the label, the more of that ingredient the food contains. In general, the fewer skipped it. If you want to lose weight, then breakfast should be a regular weapon in your weight loss arsenal. Eating breakfast:

- Boosts your metabolism first thing, which means you burn more calories throughout the morning whether you're exercising or simply sitting at your desk;
- Makes you less likely to overeat (or even binge) later in the day;

ingredients a food has the better—and the more ingredients you can identify (and pronounce), the better. Here's a quick example, using the ingredient lists of three popular whole-grain cereals:

- Cereal one: whole-grain wheat flour, malted barley flour, salt, yeast.
- Cereal two: whole-grain wheat, raisins, wheat bran, sugar, corn syrup, salt, flour, malted wheat flour.
- Cereal three: whole-grain oats, marshmallows (sugar, modified corn starch, corn syrup, dextrose, gelatin, calcium carbonate, yellows 5 & 6, blue 1, red 40, artificial flavor), sugar, oat flour, corn syrup, corn starch, salt, trisodium phosphate, color added, artificial flavor, vitamin E (mixed tocopherols) added to preserve freshness.

A quick comparison of the labels reveals that while all three start with the word "whole" in the ingredient list, the second and third cereals contain sugar (corn syrup is essentially sugar as well). Sugar is a primary ingredient of the third cereal, plus it contains added colors, flavors and "trisodium phosphate," a food additive also used in cleaning products. When you actually read the labels, you'll see foods that make similar claims on the front of the package may contain wildly different ingredients.

10 second take-away:

- Typically, the fewer ingredients (of words you can pronounce) a food contains, the better.
- When choosing a food, compare labels of similar ones to make healthier choices.

- Reduces the average number of calories you consume throughout the day;
- Gives you a better quality workout if you exercise first thing in the morning;
- Gives you more energy so you're motivated to actually exercise first thing in the morning;
- Makes you less likely to eat high-fat, high-sugar snacks mid-morning; and
- Improves your mood, making you less likely to reach for a snack to deal with anxiety or help yourself feel better.

If you need even more proof, consider these statistics from the National Weight Control Registry, a resource that tracks the habits of people who have lost at least 30 pounds and kept them

Making the Most of Your Juice

Juice is big news these days, with a wider variety than ever before. Forget the traditional juices like prune, orange, pineapple, and apple; now the shelves are teeming with açaí berry, goji berry, pomegranate, and blueberry juice—not to mention the new fruit/vegetable combo drinks that promise servings of vegetables lurking under the taste of fruit juice.

Before you gulp, keep in mind that when you can get it, whole fruit is always a better bet than juice. Ounce for ounce, whole fruit contains more fiber, fewer calories, and less sugar than fruit juice. For example, one orange contains 60 calories, 3 grams of fiber and 12 grams of sugar, while one serving (or one cup) of 100 percent orange juice can deliver twice the calories, twice the sugar, and no fiber compared to the actual orange. Plus, if you're watching your weight, fruit is more filling than juice. Liquids simply don't produce the same satiety, or feeling of fullness, that solid food does. And fruit juice is relatively high in calories.

After whole fruit, your best bet is 100 percent juice. Check the label— many "juice" drinks contain a mere 25 percent, 10 percent, or even less actual juice. Reading the label will help you confirm whether something is actually 100 percent juice, which by definition doesn't contain added off. According to the registry, 78 percent of successful "losers" eat breakfast every day, and a mere 4 percent never eat breakfast. Other long-term studies show that regular breakfast eaters tend to have a lower body mass index, or BMI (a ratio of height to weight), than those who frequently skip it or go without altogether.

BECOME A MORNING MUNCHER

So, you're convinced, or you're getting there. What's next? Change your mindset, if necessary. Quit thinking of breakfast as something that has to involve a sit-down meal of eggs, bacon, juice, toast, and coffee and start viewing it as something more flexible — even an on-the-run snack. I don't even expect you to eat first thing in the morning if you can't handle that; just get food into your body

sugars. To make it go further, dilute the juice with water or serve over ice—or look for lower-sugar, lower-calorie versions.

Don't fall for claims the "latest" juices make. All fruits contain anti-oxidants, and there's no evidence proving drinking goji berry juice (or any other) makes you healthier than people who don't drink it and eat a nutritious diet.

Finally, as for the latest fruit/vegetable juices, "reconstituted vegetable juice blend" (water mixed with concentrated juice) is the first ingredient listed, but it's not clear how much vegetables they actually contain. You're much better off actually eating your vegetables instead of drinking concentrated juice mixed with water. If you do choose vegetable juice to make up some of your veggie servings, opt for low-sodium versions—others can serve up whopping amounts of sodium.

10 second take-away:
- Whole fruit is a better bet than any juice.
- Choose 100 percent fruit juice or 100 percent low-sodium vegetable juice when you do drink juice—read the label to make sure.

within two hours of waking up. The sooner you eat something healthy, the sooner your blood sugar—and your energy, your mood, and your productivity—will go up.

Do Your Body Good with the Right Kind of Dairy

According to mypyramid.com, the USDA's website to help Americans eat healthier, you should aim for three servings of dairy products every day. Dairy products provide protein, calcium, and other nutrients, but full-fat dairy foods are also loaded with saturated fat—bad news for your heart and waistline. Your best bet for dairy options is to choose organic (hormone- and antibiotic-free) when you can. Look for the "USDA Organic" seal on the label to ensure your milk is free of added growth and reproductive hormones. Choose lower-fat products, like one percent or skim (fat-free) milk over whole (full-fat) or two percent. A cup of two percent milk contains about 140 calories and 5 grams of fat, while a cup of skim milk contains about 90 calories and less than 1 gram of fat.

If you're lactose-intolerant or don't like dairy foods, aim for three servings of calcium-rich foods each day. Foods like calcium-fortified soy milk, calcium-fortified orange juice, legumes, leafy green vegetables, tortillas made with limestone, tofu, nuts, and fish like sardines and salmon that contain bones are all good sources of calcium.

But there's much more to dairy than milk. You may be surprised to learn I do recommend full-fat cheeses—they taste better (so you can often eat less and feel more satisfied) and they are less processed than fat-free or low-fat versions. A serving of cheese is 1 ounce (about the size of two dice). As with all dairy, buy organic cheeses when possible.

When it comes to yogurt you have a slew of choices, but many aren't that great. With yogurt, you especially need to read the Nutrition Facts label. Check the following:

- Calorie count. One serving of yogurt could include a mere 70 calories but go all the way up to 250. If you're watching your

Breakfast at Home

Half the battle is simply getting into the breakfast habit. While variety is a good thing, it may be easier to eat the same breakfast most mornings. If you're stressed by trying to make it out of the house in the morning, make it easy on yourself. If you have time for a simple meal of high-fiber cereal with skim milk or soy milk

weight, pick yogurts with 150 calories or less per one-cup serving.

- Sugar content. Plain yogurt doesn't contain added sugars, but many fruit-flavored varieties have added sugar (often as "high fructose corn syrup") and can deliver 40 or more grams of sugar (20 or more grams of that as added sugar) per one-cup serving. (Better bet? Choose nonfat, plain yogurt and add honey or fresh fruit for sweetness and additional flavor.)

- Organic—or not? Just as you don't want added sugars, you want to avoid added colors and flavors, too. Who needs them? Organic yogurt contains no extra ingredients and is produced without antibiotics, pesticides, or growth hormones.

- Live active cultures. The phrase "live active cultures" on the label tells you the yogurt contains probiotics that help support your digestive tract and may boost your immune function as well. (You may also see names like bifudus, s. thermophilus, l. acidolophilus, or l. casei on the label.)

- Try Greek yogurt. Go for an all-natural Greek yogurt (e.g., Chobani, FAGE Total, or StonyField OIKIS) for a creamier taste. Greek yogurt contains twice the protein as regular yogurt to keep you feeling full longer, and the varieties listed here have no artificial flavors or preservatives.

10 second take-away:
- Choose all-natural, organic dairy products when you can.
- Opt for nonfat or low-fat dairy products and limit added sugars.

most mornings, you'll meet your nutritional and energy needs with a minimum of fuss. Who cares if you're eating the same thing?

Here are seven at-home breakfast options:

- *Oatmeal yum.* Top 1 cup of plain oatmeal with 2 tablespoons each of chopped nuts and dried fruit, a pinch of cinnamon, and a drizzle of honey.
- *"Egg-lish" muffin crostini & cheese.* Put 1 poached egg, 1 slice of lean ham, and 1 thin (1/2 ounce) slice of Swiss cheese on a 1/2 toasted whole-wheat English muffin.
- *B&B bruschetta.* Top 1 slice of whole-wheat toast with 1 tablespoon of all-natural nut butter, 1/2 sliced banana, and a drizzle of honey.
- *Cereal & fruit.* Pour 1 cup of skim milk (or calcium-fortified soy milk) over 1 cup of high-fiber, whole-grain cereal and serve with 1/2 pink or red grapefruit on the side.
- *Waffle wise.* Toast 2 low-fat whole-grain frozen waffles with 1/2 cup fresh (or thawed, unsweetened frozen) berries and 1 tablespoon of maple syrup.
- *"Egg-lish" muffin & greens.* Stuff 1 whole-wheat English muffin with 1 cooked egg, 1 slice of cooked Canadian bacon, watercress or baby spinach, and a squirt of lemon.
- *Cheese toast.* Top a slice of whole-wheat toast with 1 slice of part-skim mozzarella cheese with a few fresh basil leaves; serve with 1 cup low-sodium 100 percent vegetable juice (add a few drops of hot sauce for eye-opening pizzazz).

On the Run

If the concept of a sit-down morning meal makes you laugh, then plan on taking something with you to work to eat during your commute, or in the car. (Same goes for moms doing the school run.) You may spend a minute (probably less), but you'll get that time back during your day, through higher energy levels and an improved ability to get things done.

Real People, Real Breakfasts—and Real Results

We know Alyssa, who was quoted at the beginning of this chapter, has the breakfast thing down. Here's how other people make "munch every morn" work, even with little time:

> I keep oatmeal at work. Sometimes I'm running late and have to wait until I get to work to eat, but that's better than missing it altogether. By eating breakfast, I oftentimes eat less at lunch. Sometimes I just snack after lunch instead of having a full meal. Breakfast really carries me through the day more than lunch, and there's no after-lunch crash either.
>
> —Jessica, 37, college instructor

> After being diagnosed as hypoglycemic, I started eating breakfast regularly. My life changed completely. Suddenly I had more energy, stopped getting the afternoon "brain fog", ate less throughout the day. Breakfast is hard, especially because I travel a lot for work. I've been known to bring pre-portioned bags of almonds or even hard boiled eggs with me (protein bars have too much sugar for a hypoglycemic), and am delighted by how well they travel.
>
> —Stacey, 46, consultant

> Breakfast used to be rushed, or skipped entirely. Now, my husband and I make a point to have a hot breakfast every day (water, eggs, cheese, oatmeal, grapefruit, etc.) I'm more alert, thinner, and generally feel much better. Make the time to get up a few minutes earlier in order to sit quietly and have breakfast each day. Things like muffin batter, baked oatmeal, and hard boiled eggs can be made at any time and kept in the refrigerator for the next morning.
>
> —Cassandra, 38, transportation planner

Milk it for All Its Worth

When you think of milk, you probably visualize cow's milk, but other options are available if you need them. While other "milks" may not be as high in calcium as cow's milk is (containing 300 mg per one-cup serving; or about 30 percent of your Daily Value), manufacturers usually add calcium (and sometimes vitamin D) to make their products similar to cow's milk. Vitamin D is important because it helps you absorb calcium in the milk and has recently been shown to help prevent a number of chronic diseases. Here's the rundown on other popular milks:

- Lactose-free milk. This is actually regular cow's milk with a twist—the lactose has already been digested so it won't create stomach problems if you're sensitive. This beverage contains the same number of calories and calcium as regular milk.
- Soy milk. If you can't tolerate cow's milk or prefer a vegan option, soy milk is a great choice. Made from pressed soybeans, a one-cup serving contains about 100 to 140 calories. Soy milk is naturally lower in protein and calcium than cow's milk; most makers add calcium. Though higher in fat than skim milk, it also contains omega-3 fats, which are good for heart health.
- Almond milk. Did you know milk can be produced from finely ground almonds and water? This thin milk has no saturated fat, but little protein—about a gram per one-cup serving. Manufacturers typically add calcium and vitamin D, but check the label to be sure what you're getting.
- Rice milk. This milk made from rice and water is low in protein. Makers add calcium and vitamin D. It contains no saturated fat.
- Coconut milk. Derived from the flesh of the coconut, coconut milk is typically high in calories and saturated fat, but its fat contains a type of MCFAs, or medium-chain fatty acids, that may offer health benefits. Look for "light" coconut milk drinks with fewer calories and less fat.

10 second take-away:

- Read labels to make sure your alternative milk contains calcium and vitamin D.
- Choose low-fat or fat-free "milk" products and remember to limit your portion size to one-cup servings.

Here are seven speedy options you can bring along:

- **Berry smoothie**. Blend 1 cup of low-fat Greek yogurt, 1/2 cup berries, 1/2 cup of 100 percent apple juice, and 1/2 cup of crushed ice until smooth.
- **Greek yogurt & jam**. Mix 1/2 cup of low-fat Greek yogurt with 1 tablespoon of 100 percent fruit spread or jam of your choice.
- **Bar it**. Bring along 1 whole-food bar [See Sidebar, Get the Most Energy from Your Energy Bar, on page 107] and 1 can (5.5 ounce) low-sodium 100 percent vegetable juice.
- **Muffin & juice**. Bring along 1 high-fiber fruit and nut muffin and 1 cup of 100 percent fruit juice in a reusable container.
- **Energy pita**. Top 1/2 whole-grain pita with Neufchatel (light cream) cheese, 2 tablespoons of chopped nuts and 2 tablespoons of dried fruit.
- **Egg sandwich**. Place a scrambled or sliced hard-boiled egg with a cheese slice and leafy greens (like arugula) on a whole-grain roll.
- **Yogurt parfait**. Mix 1 ounce of granola and 1/2 cup of seasonal fruit of your choice into 1 cup of nonfat plain yogurt.

Restaurant Options

Eating breakfast out? Here are seven options if you're traveling or eating breakfast at a restaurant:

- **Eggs of the border**. Have 1 to 2 scrambled eggs with 1/2 cup of black beans, 2 slices of avocado, and lots of salsa.
- **Egg, toast, fruit**. Have 1 scrambled or hard-boiled egg with 1 slice of whole-wheat toast and 1 piece of fresh fruit.
- **Oatmeal plus**. Add 1 tablespoon nut butter to 1 cup of plain oatmeal; have a side of seasonal fresh fruit.
- **Veggie omelet**. Wrap 1 medium vegetable omelet in a whole-wheat tortilla, or have the omelet with 1 slice of whole-wheat bread.
- **Egg sandwich**. Have 1 toasted English muffin with 1 egg and 1 slice of lean meat or cheese.

- *Cereal & fruit*. Pour 1 cup of skim milk (or calcium-fortified soy milk) over 1 cup of high-fiber cereal, and have 1 small banana with it.
- *Poached eggs on greens*. Serve 2 poached eggs on a bed of steamed spinach; sprinkle with lemon juice, and enjoy with 1 slice of whole-grain toast with 100 percent fruit jam.

The News About Morning Brews

I've got good news for you. If you can't face the idea of giving up your morning cup of coffee—you don't have to. Plenty of research shows that in moderate doses (say, a cup or two), coffee increases mental alertness and improves mood—and coffee in the morning isn't likely to affect your sleep pattern at night.

But there's something even better than coffee when it comes to health—tea, the most popular beverage in the world. Hundreds of research studies show tea's health benefits. Tea is linked with everything from better heart health to improved immune function to increasing your metabolism. Tea contains antioxidants called flavanoids, that help protect your body against free radicals. (Free radicals cause cellular damage and appear to up your risk of developing conditions like heart disease and cancer.)

In addition to caffeine, tea also contains an amino acid called l-theanine that creates a feeling of calm alertness—which is just what you need when you're stressed and on the go. In fact, I'd say given the choice between tea and water, tea is an even better choice because of its antioxidant boost.

If you drink your coffee or tea "straight up," (i.e., no added cream, sugar, or other ingredients), it's also calorie-free. But if you prefer lattes, mochas, or frappuccinos, you may be in trouble calorie-wise. A "grande" (small) mocha frappuccino blended coffee at Starbucks contains 260 calories while a small latte contains 190 calories. Larger drinks and higher-sugar versions can contain twice that.

While a cup of black coffee contains no calories or fat, cream and sugar sure do. Just 1 tablespoon of sugar contains 45 calories, and

Now that you're armed with strategies to become a morning muncher for life, you're ready to tackle the next meal of the day: lunch. Read on to learn to make the most of the noon-time meal.

1 tablespoon of powdered cream can contain 25 to 60 calories while 2 tablespoons of liquid creamer can range from 15 to 85 calories. To put that in perspective, if your coffee "accessories" add up to an extra 100 calories a day, that's equivalent to adding an extra 10 pounds a year. Your best bet is to add skim milk and 1 tablespoon or less of sugar per cup.

While a little bit of caffeine can help improve mental alertness and mood, you can have too much of a good thing. A typical cup of brewed coffee has about 133 grams of caffeine, while a grande brewed coffee at Starbucks has 320 grams. The same size at Dunkin' Donuts has 206 grams of caffeine. Tea contains less caffeine—a cup of brewed tea has about 53 grams of caffeine while a Snapple Lemon tea has about 100 grams. Most sodas have about 50 grams of caffeine per 12-ounce can while one 8-ounce can of Red Bull has about 80 grams.

People develop tolerance to caffeine over time. In other words, the more caffeine you consume regularly, the less impact it may have. Everyday caffeine consumption of 300 mg or more can dehydrate you, cause stomach problems, or cause headaches from withdrawal when you don't consume your usual amount. If you notice these kinds of symptoms, gradually reduce your intake to reduce your reliance on it to get through the day.

10 second take-away:
- Choose tea when possible, for its health benefits.
- Remember that coffee drinks can be high in calories. Brewed coffee is a better choice.

4

NOONTIME NOSHING:

Eat-on-the-Run Lunch Options

66 My biggest lunch issue is speed. This meal has to be quick, in
between my classes, and if I have to go off-campus for lunch
it puts me in a fast food drive-thru line. So I do go there
sometimes, but often just get a sandwich and skip the fries. 99

—Jessica, 37, college instructor

Does Jessica's biggest lunch challenge—the need for speed—
ring a bell? Do you sometimes skip lunch to save time, or realize
at 3 p.m. you forgot to eat? Do you scatter crumbs on your laptop
while munching a sandwich and catching up on email? Whether
you work outside the home or not, finding time for lunch—let
alone a healthy one—is a major challenge for most people. Yet
the busier you are, the more you need the nutrients and energy a
healthy lunch provides.

Portion Patrol: They're Smaller Than You Think

Think you can identify a "normal" portion? Probably not. Studies show we routinely overestimate the size of a regular portion and underestimate our caloric intake. Here's a guide to typical portion sizes and how large they actually are:

Grains

1 serving of cereal = 1 cup = baseball (or your fist)

1 serving of cooked rice, pasta, or mashed potato = 1/2 cup = 2 golf balls

1 serving of rolls or small starch portions = 2/3 cup = tennis ball

1 serving of bread = 1 ounce = 1 slice

Fruits/Vegetables

1 serving of fruit or vegetables = 1 cup = baseball (or your fist)

1 serving of dried fruit or vegetables = 1/4 cup = golf ball

Dairy Products

1 serving of cheese = 1 ounce = 2 dice

1 serving of milk or yogurt = 1 cup = baseball (or your fist)

Beans/Nuts

1 serving of beans = 1/2 cup = 2 golf balls

1 serving of nuts = 1/4 cup = golf ball

1 serving of nut butter = 2 tablespoons = ping pong ball (or 2 poker chips)

Meats/Fish/Poultry

1 serving of meat, fish or poultry = 3 ounces = deck of cards (or a checkbook)

Fats/Oils

1 serving of oil or butter = 1 tablespoon = poker chip (or your thumb tip)

BROWN-BAGGING IT

The simplest option, when you're on the go or at work, is to bring your own. Making your own lunch may take a little extra time in the morning, but it's based on several smart concepts. First, you can bring foods you like, control portion size, and you know what you're eating. You also have something healthy to eat so you don't end up starving and making less-than-healthy choices (vending machine, anyone?). And you'll save money, too.

A healthy lunch can be a sandwich made with lean meat, plus veggies and a piece of fruit. Including protein (the meat) and fiber (the whole-grain bread, veggies, and fruit) provides the elements for a satisfying meal. In the next section, I'll give you shopping tips so you know what to keep on hand for healthy lunches.

Experiment with different types of bread, meat, and veggies if you're a sandwich person. Replace your usual ham and Swiss on rye with thinly sliced roast beef on pumpernickel bread, a variety of veggies (e.g., sweet onion, watercress, thinly sliced cucumber, shredded carrot and/or tomato) and spicy mustard. Or make tortilla wraps by spreading a thin layer of cream cheese on a whole-wheat tortilla and adding lower-fat ham, cheese, or turkey, and vegetables like green or red peppers, onions, broccoli, cucumbers, and tomatoes. Some grilled chicken and vegetables, pesto sauce and a little low-fat mayonnaise wrapped in a whole-wheat tortilla are just as delicious as the popular fast food variety—and better for you, too.

Brown-bagging isn't boredom if you mix it up now and then. Here are seven lunch options to carry with you and eat at work:

- *Tuna hummus dip.* Mix together 1/2 cup of canned, drained water-packed albacore tuna with 2 tablespoons of hummus and a splash of lemon juice; eat with slices of celery or cucumber or a few baked pita chips.

- *Italian bean salad.* Toss 1 can of drained white beans with 1 teaspoon each of balsamic vinegar and extra-virgin olive oil and add fresh herbs (e.g, parsley, basil and/or oregano) to taste.

- *Frozen burrito.* Heat an Amy's organic frozen burrito and top with lots of fresh salsa and 1/2 cup of low-fat cottage cheese.

- *Mini Italian sub.* Place 1 ounce (2 slices) of prosciutto or lean

ham, 1 ounce part-skim mozzarella, 1 teaspoon 100 percent
apricot spread, and a large handful of fresh baby greens like
baby arugula on a whole-grain roll. Enjoy with seasonal fresh
fruit or 1/4 cup of dried vegetables.

- *Frozen entrée.* Choose a healthy frozen entrée [See Sidebar,
  Frozen Meals: Making the Best Choice, on page 68], organic
  if possible, and serve with a side of seasonal fresh fruit or 1
  cup of low-fat Greek yogurt.

- *Turkey sandwich.* Place 3 slices (3 ounces) of turkey meat and
  1 slice of reduced-fat cheese (organic if possible) on 2 slices of

Shaking Off the Salt

How much salt do you eat? Chances are, you consume more than
you think. The recommended sodium intake for adults is 2,400 mg a
day, which sounds like a lot until you realize how much hidden salt is in
the food you eat. A large burger at a fast food restaurant may contain
1,200 mg of sodium. A can of soup may have more than 1,000 mg, while
a small can of vegetable juice can give you 650 mg of sodium. In fact,
77 percent of your daily salt intake probably comes not from the shaker,
but from processed foods.

While you may think of foods like French fries and nuts as high in
salt, processed foods often contain much more. You don't notice it,
because you don't taste it the way you taste the salt on a handful of
nuts or a couple of French fries. One ounce of roasted, salted nuts has
about 100 mg of sodium, but because the salt is on the outside of the
nuts, it hits your taste buds first, giving you the salty flavor.

While we tend to use "sodium" and "salt" interchangeably, salt refers
to the dietary mineral found naturally in some foods. Sodium chloride,
or table salt, is the salt that raises your risk of health problems, including
high blood pressure, and is the one you want to limit. Even if your blood
pressure is normal, new research shows keeping your salt intake low
can help your arteries stay healthy and reduce your risk of developing
heart disease or having a stroke sometime in the future. Need a more
immediate reason to cut back? Too much salt can also cause you to
retain water and feel bloated.

whole-grain bread and 1 tablespoon of Dijon mustard; enjoy with 1 piece of seasonal fresh fruit or 1 cup of low-fat Greek yogurt.

- **Soup's on.** Serve 2 cups of a low-sodium soup with beans and vegetables with 5 whole-grain crackers and 1 seasonal fresh fruit.

EATING AT HOME BEGINS AT THE STORE

This sounds like the perfect environment. By eating at home you can control what you eat, when you eat, and how much, right? That's true—as long as you have healthy options on hand. That's why I'll give you four smart tips for shopping on the run.

But while too much salt is a bad thing, consuming less than 500 mg per day isn't healthy either. Sodium works with potassium to help regulate fluid balance in the body. Sodium is also essential for proper nerve function, metabolizing proteins and carbohydrates, and maintaining the body's acid/alkali balance, which is important for overall health. But not all salt is nutritionally equal—choose kosher or sea salt as both contain natural minerals and slightly less sodium content than regular table salt.

To lower your sodium intake, read the Nutrition Facts label on foods to check how much sodium they contain. Aim for less than 2,400 mg per day. Eat fewer processed foods and more fresh food that's naturally low in sodium. If you do buy processed foods like soup, vegetable juice, and frozen dinners, look for low-sodium versions and cut back on the amount of condiments you use. Ketchup, mustard, relish, and salad dressings all contain sodium. Using a variety of spices and herbs can help add flavor to your food without the extra sodium your body doesn't need. And remember the taste for salt is learned—which means once you get used to eating less, you won't miss it.

10 second take-away:

- Limit your salt intake to 2,400 mg a day or less by reading the Nutrition Facts label. Choose kosher or sea salt, as both contain natural minerals and slightly less sodium than table salt.
- Choose fresh foods over processed to reduce your salt intake.

On-the-Run Shopping Strategy #1: Plan Ahead

You need a plan—or at least a list. Head to the store without one and you'll waste time and money you don't have, and feel overwhelmed by the variety of eye-catching, high-sugar, high-fat, processed foods that sabotage your weight. Keep a notepad in your kitchen to write down foods you know you need, and have a snack before you go. Shop hungry and you'll be amazed at the chips, ice cream, and cookies that somehow leap into your cart.

Frozen Meals—Making the Best Choice

Frozen entrees can make a great option for a quick meal. Keep a few in your fridge at home or toss one in the break room refrigerator at work and you'll have a meal in minutes.

However, not all frozen meals are created equal. Many are high in fat, calories, and sodium so pay close attention to the labels on precooked entrees and other convenience foods. You want entrees that contain protein and fiber and aren't too high in fat, sodium, and artificial ingredients. A good rule of thumb for frozen entrees is to choose items with less than 10 grams of total fat and less than 5 grams of saturated fat. Look for entrees that contain under 500 mg of sodium. If the entrée has more than one serving, be sure to multiply the numbers if you eat the entire thing. And as I've mentioned before, the fewer ingredients with complicated or hard-to-pronounce names a food has, the better.

Some brands are made with all-organic foods. Although these may be a little more expensive, if you find a brand you like (many of my clients swear by Amy's), you know you're getting a high-quality, nutritious meal even when you're on the run.

10 second take-away:

- Look for frozen meals with less than 10 grams of total fat and 500 mg of sodium.
- Choose frozen meals that contain plenty of vegetables and at least 3 grams of fiber to boost your lunch's nutritional content.

On-the-Run Shopping Strategy #2:
Run to the Borders

Ever wonder why dairy products are always found at the back of the supermarket? This forces you to walk through the entire store even if you've only come for a gallon of milk. Marketers know you'll wind up grabbing other items along the way. The basics of your healthy diet—fruits and veggies, lean protein sources, low-fat dairy products, and whole-grains—are found on the edges of the store, and that's where you should spend most of your shopping time.

The produce section is located in the front of most stores, so begin your shopping trip with fruits and veggies. Here's a good rule of thumb: different nutrients and antioxidants produce different colors, so the more color you have in your grocery cart, the better. Make it a habit to pick up three or more colors on each trip you make to the store: some greens (like spinach, broccoli, cucumbers), reds (tomatoes, apples, plums), yellows (squash, yellow peppers, bananas), oranges (oranges, sweet potatoes), purples (eggplant, red cabbage), and whites (onions, garlic).

On-the-Run Shopping Strategy #3:
Read All About It

Usually people shop by grabbing what looks good or what's on sale. Become a label reader and you'll get the most nutrients for your buck. For example, in the meat section, look for packaging that says "higher than 90% lean" or "95% extra lean." Those are the lowest-fat meat choices. If the label doesn't have a "lean" designation, it's probably high in fat. Also examine the cut of meat itself. The more marbling you see in the meat, the higher the fat content. Good lean meat choices include sirloin steak, skirt steak, pork tenderloin, and chicken and turkey—but check the label as ground turkey can be higher in fat than expected. Whenever you can, choose organic, grass-fed meats and poultry to reduce your exposure to hormones and pesticides [See Sidebar, The Big O, on this page.] For the healthiest diet overall, aim to eat red meat about once a week, poultry and fish a few times a week, and choose plant-based meals the rest of the time. You'll cut fat intake and increase your intake of fruits, veggies, and legumes.

In the dairy section, skip the whole milk and full-fat yogurt in favor of one percent or skim versions. If you're accustomed to the full-fat flavor, give yourself about two weeks for your taste buds to

The Big O: What is Organic—and Is it Worth the Expense?

Let's talk organic. Is organic food really better for you? Is it worth the extra expense? And what does organic actually signify?

First, "organic" means food has been grown and processed without the use of synthetic fertilizers, pesticides, genetic engineering, or irradiation. A package or label that reads "certified organic" means it was grown according to uniform standards verified by independent state or private organizations. To claim "certified organic" status companies must maintain certain records, allow their farms and processing facilities to be inspected, and undergo soil and water tests that ensure these standards are maintained.

Don't be tricked into thinking a food that claims to be "natural" is also organic. According to the USDA, a food can be called "natural" if it's minimally processed and doesn't contain artificial flavoring or coloring, chemical preservatives, or artificial or synthetic ingredients. That means foods can be called "natural" regardless of whether organic standards were met.

When you eat organic, you know you're getting food free from pesticides and other additives, but organics may promise another benefit as well. Research shows some types of organic produce contain higher levels of certain vitamins and phytochemicals (substances found in plants that help fight disease) than their conventional counterparts. For example, one study found that organically grown oranges contained more vitamin C and produced more antioxidant activity than non-organic oranges. Another study found organic grapes contained more polyphenols (substances found in plants that appear adjust and you won't notice the difference. Choose organic dairy foods when possible. Read the labels on cheese and yogurt [See Sidebar, Do Your Body Good, on page 54] so you know what you're getting, and do the same with canned soups and vegetables, which tend to be high in sodium. [See Sidebar, Shaking Off the Salt, on page 66.] And don't forget to stock up on wholesome carb choices. Whole-grain breads and pastas (remember to look for the word

to have antioxidant properties), and resveratrol, a plant-produced substance that helps fight off disease.

While some organic foods may provide more nutrients for your buck, these foods do tend to cost more than conventionally-grown versions. But even with the recent recession, a marketing company survey found nearly fifty percent of us purchase as much or more organic food as before the recession. If you worry about your budget, go organic with foods that are most likely to be tainted by pesticides. Or check out your local farmers market. Relying on family farms and local growers can save you money and help save the planet, too.

If you can't opt for all organic, all the time, spend your money on organic dairy and meat to reduce your exposure to hormones that are often added to conventionally-raised cattle and other animals. Because some fruits and vegetables (called the "dirty dozen") are more likely to be loaded with pesticides, you're better off choosing organic apples, pears, nectarines, peaches, strawberries, cherries, grapes, carrots, celery, bell peppers, tomatoes and lettuce.

10 second take-away:

- Visit farmers markets for locally-grown organic produce. Prioritize and focus on the "dirty dozen," which are more likely to be loaded with pesticides.
- When possible, buy organic dairy foods and meats to reduce your exposure to antibiotics and hormones.

"whole" on the label as the first ingredient) with at least two grams of fiber per serving are your best bet.

On-the-Run Shopping Strategy #4: Check Your Cart

Before you leave the store, take a look at your cart. At a minimum, it should contain a selection of produce, lean protein, low-fat dairy products, and whole-grains. That doesn't mean your cart can't include any "treats"—but be smart. If you love ice cream, buy portion-controlled ice cream cups or bars instead of a half-gallon of ice cream. Yes, it's more expensive, but you'll be able to maintain smaller (and lower-calorie) portions. For a healthier sweet treat, go for frozen 100 percent fruit bars.

Good and Not-So-Good Seafood: What You Need to Know About Mercury

You know fish and seafood are good for you, because they're typically high in protein, low in fat, and contain omega-3 fats linked with heart health. Yet some fish is better than others, at least when it comes to the amount of mercury it contains.

Mercury is a metal found in the environment, but if you ingest too much your body takes a long time to get rid of it. Excess mercury can harm the brains of young children and developing fetuses. (To be safe, if you're pregnant or trying to get pregnant, ask your doctor whether you should avoid all seafood or which ones are safe.)

Fish absorb mercury through the water they live in, and when you eat fish and seafood, you absorb this mercury as well. Most fish contain small amounts of mercury, but others contain significantly more. The US Food and Drug Administration recommends women who are pregnant or trying to become pregnant, nursing mothers, and young children avoid all fish that is high in mercury, including king mackerel, shark, swordfish, and tilefish. They can eat up to 12 ounces per week of fish that is lower in mercury, such as canned light tuna, catfish, pollock, salmon, and shrimp. Albacore, or white tuna has more mercury than

Once you've mastered the grocery store, you're ready to make delicious, quick lunches at home. Here are seven handy options:

- *Margarita melt.* Toast 1 whole-grain English muffin and top each side with marinara sauce and 2-3 tablespoons of shredded, part-skim mozzarella and heat in microwave until cheese melts. Top with fresh basil and serve with a side of seasonal fresh fruit.
- *Bean dip burrito.* Combine 1/4 cup black bean dip with 2 tablespoons of store-prepared guacamole. Wrap in a whole-wheat tortilla with sliced grape tomatoes and chopped Romaine lettuce.
- *Sweet potato delight.* Microwave a medium sweet potato and top with plain low-fat Greek yogurt and a drizzle of maple syrup or

canned light tuna, and tuna steaks have more mercury than canned tuna.

According to the American Heart Association, people should eat at least two servings weekly of lake herring, lake trout, mackerel, salmon, sardines, or tuna for the healthy omega-3 fats they contain. But if you're a woman who could get pregnant (even if you're not actively trying to), it's smart to follow the mercury recommendations when choosing what kind of fish you'll have for supper. Easier yet, visit the Environmental Defense Fund's website, www.edf.org, for a printable Seafood Pocket Guide and a Sushi Pocket Guide you can carry with you.

10 second take-away:
- Aim for two servings a week of omega-3 rich fish like lake herring, lake trout, mackerel, salmon, sardines, or canned light tuna.
- Avoid fish that is high in mercury like king mackerel, shark, swordfish, and tilefish, especially if you're trying to get pregnant (or even if it's a possibility).

teaspoon of orange marmalade; enjoy with 2 slices of lean ham, rolled.

- *Caribbean avocado dip*. Mash 1/2 of a soft avocado with a cup of nonfat plain Greek yogurt, the juice of half a lime and hot pepper sauce to taste; eat with 3 ounces of shrimp (about 14 medium shrimp) or a handful of baked plantain chips.
- *Energy pita*. Spread 1/2 whole-grain pita with Neufchatel (light cream) cheese and top with 2 tablespoons each of chopped nuts and dried fruit.
- *Egg sandwich*. Place a scrambled or sliced hard-boiled egg with a slice of natural, reduced-fat cheese and leafy greens (like arugula) on a whole-grain roll.

Fast Facts on Fat

Several years ago, the big news about fat focused on trans fats, hydrogenated oils that appeared to boost the risk of heart disease even more than saturated fat. Today, manufacturers have eliminated most trans fats from the food supply, but you still have to make smart choices when it comes to choosing fats.

Saturated fats—the ones found in animal products and some vegetable oils like palm and coconut—are most likely to raise your risk of heart disease. "Good" fats like monounsaturated and polyunsaturated fats can help lower your risk of heart disease by decreasing your LDL, or bad cholesterol levels. Nuts, seeds, avocados, olive oil, peanut oil, and canola oil are all good sources of monounsaturated fat, while vegetable oils like safflower oil, corn oil, sunflower oil, nuts and seeds, and soy oil all contain polyunsaturated fats. Omega-3 fats, found in foods like herring, mackerel, salmon, flaxseeds, flaxseed oil, and walnuts, are a specific type of polyunsaturated fats that are good for heart and brain function.

Fat not only tastes good—it takes longer to digest, so it's more satiating (meaning it will ward off hunger longer) than eating carbs or protein on their own, though protein is satiating too. But because fat is higher in calories (9 calories a gram) than carbs or protein (each of

- *Yogurt parfait*. Add 1 ounce of granola and 1/2 cup of seasonal fresh fruit of choice to a cup of nonfat plain yogurt.

SURVIVING THE LUNCH CHALLENGE:
FAST FOOD DOESN'T HAVE TO MAKE YOU FAT

We've talked about bringing your own and eating at home, but chances are, much of your lunchtime noshing is on a "grab-and-go" basis, whether from a fast food restaurant or deli counter. You're more likely to zip through the drive-thru window than have a sit-down lunch, which ups the challenge when it comes to eating well. In the next chapter we'll discuss dinner and talk more about sit-down restaurants.

which has 4 calories a gram) and is relatively dense, when you eat too much of it, your waistline will suffer.

However, fat is an essential part of your healthy diet. The current recommendations for healthy adults are to aim for 25 to 30 percent of your calories to come from fat (or about 55-65 grams a day for a 2,000 calorie diet), with only one-third of that coming from saturated fat (or about 18-21 grams a day for a 2,000 calorie diet). Consume more omega-3 fats in your diet and cut back on the saturated and fatty processed foods you consume. In addition, reducing your intake of refined carbohydrates can help lower your triglyceride levels, which is good news for your heart.

10 second take-away:
- Cut back on the amount of animal products you consume and choose leaner options to reduce your intake of saturated fat.
- Opt for nuts, seeds, and vegetable oils like safflower, corn, olive, flaxseed, and sunflower and fatty fish like herring, mackerel and salmon to include healthy monounsaturated and polyunsaturated fats into your diet.

What can you do? First, forget about your monetary budget and think of your caloric budget instead. In other words, don't supersize your meal, even if you get double the amount of food for a few pennies more. Go for normal portions. A McDonald's hamburger and small fries clocks in at 480 calories and 21.5 grams of fat. Choose a Big Mac and large fries instead and you'll take in a whopping 960 calories and 54 grams of fat.

Let me say something about fast food. Sure, it's cheap—but it costs you in the long run. Americans spend 40 billion dollars a year on diet products and programs to try to lose weight—much of which comes from cheap, overly plentiful food. The irony! You save money on food in the short run, but spend money trying

Drinks with Your Diet in Mind

You already learned about the dangers of alcohol: imbibing makes you more likely to overeat and slip off your healthy eating plan. But I realize most people want to enjoy an alcoholic beverage occasionally. That's fine, as long as you keep in mind that we can make smart choices, or not-so-smart ones. Beers are now available with less than 70 calories, but in general, a beer or glass of wine contains between 100 and 150 calories. Remember, too, that the size of the glass and serving makes a big difference. A single "glass" of wine may actually be two servings.

Drink a glass of water, sparkling water, or tea between drinks to slow your consumption and stay hydrated. Yes, these are liquid calories, but they do add up fast.

Research suggests moderate drinking may have some heart-protective effects. But what is moderate? Just one drink a day for women, and two drinks a day for men. Drink more than that on a regular basis and you not only consume unnecessary calories, you also increase your risk of high blood pressure, stroke, some cancers, and other conditions. And sorry, but you can't save up your daily drinks and have them all on the weekend. Your metabolism doesn't work that way.

To be healthy and fit, follow moderate drinking guidelines and keep this caloric comparison of popular drinks in mind:

to get the weight off, not to mention the time and stress dieting entails. That's why I'd rather have you pay more for healthier food now than throw away time and money in the future trying to lose weight. And don't forget the money you may spend on higher medical bills due to poorer health during the rest of your life.

While fast food is convenient, fast, and cheap, most is high in fat and calories, deficient in complex carbohydrates and nutrients. No surprise that the more frequently we eat fast food, the more likely we are to take in more calories, more fat, and less fiber than people who frequent the Golden Arches less often. Fortunately most fast food chains have expanded their menus to include at least a few healthier choices, such as grilled meat, baked potatoes, and salads.

Drink	Serving size/ounces	calories
Beer	12	150
"Light" beer	12	110
Dark beer	12	168
Spirits (Scotch, vodka, gin)	1.5	100
Red wine	5	105
White wine	5	100
Sparkling wine	5	106
Mixed drinks (on average):		
Bloody Mary	7	87
Cosmopolitan	4	213
Gin and tonic	6	143
Margarita	6	278
Martini	2.2	135
Screwdriver	7	208

10 second take-away:

- Limit your alcoholic consumption to one drink a day for women and two for men—or at least drink a glass of water or other nonalcoholic beverage for every "drink."
- Choose light beer or wine, which has the fewest calories/drink.

But expect to pay extra for the healthier choices.

Skip the soda, or at least get diet. Better yet, order water, low-fat milk, or unsweetened tea If you're at a deli, sub shop, or pizza place, you can still find healthier options. For example, ordering thin-crust pizza with "easy" (i.e., light) cheese and fresh vegetables is a much better choice than a deep-dish sausage and pepperoni pie. While I'm sure that's no surprise to you, the degree of difference shocks most of my clients. For example, a slice of thin-crust veggie pizza is about 200 calories and 7 grams of fat, while a slice of deep-

Most Popular = Most Fattening.

A recent survey revealed what you may have already suspected: many of the most popular choices at restaurants tend to be the highest in fat and calories. Here are the most often-featured dishes at restaurants and the percentage of customers who order them:

Appetizers

Chicken wings - 46 percent
Chicken strips/fingers - 42 percent
Onion rings - 33 percent
Mozzarella sticks - 33 percent
French fries - 32 percent

Notice anything? That's right—every single one of the most popular appetizers are fried. That's a lot of fat and calories, and only the beginning of your meal. As an alternative, turn your appetizer into an AppeSizer by choosing salsa or hummus and fresh vegetables, a small dinner salad with dressing on the side, a shrimp cocktail, or a bowl of broth-based soup.

Here are the most popular dishes in other categories—and note how few of them are healthy choices:

Red meat entrees

Rib-eye steak - 38 percent
Filet mignon - 38 percent
Strip steak - 32 percent

deep pizza packs in 480 calories and 26 grams of fat. That's a big difference, especially when you consider that most people eat more than one slice. A roast beef or Italian beef sandwich is a leaner, lighter choice than pastrami, ham, or salami. Skip the mayonnaise and other high-fat sauces in favor of mustard and ketchup.

Again, watch your portion size. That sandwich may actually be two or three sizes larger than normal. Choose whole-grain bread over white, and top with low-calorie, nutritionally dense vegetables like green peppers, tomatoes, onions, lettuce, and

Pork ribs - 28 percent
Prime rib/sirloin steak (tie) - 27 percent

Soups

Clam or seafood chowder - 39 percent
French onion - 36 percent
Tomato - 34 percent
Chicken noodle - 33 percent
Vegetable - 29 percent

Salads

Caesar - 66 percent
Caesar with chicken/shrimp - 60 percent
Tossed green salad - 54 percent
Coleslaw - 37 percent
Cobb salad - 30 percent

With the exception of several soups and the tossed green salad, the most popular restaurant choices are also the most fattening. I'm not saying you can't eat out and still maintain a healthy weight, but keep in mind that it's up to you to make the most of your selections, watch your portions, and avoid overeating.

pickles. Stuffing your sandwich with vegetables will help fill you up and boost your nutrient intake. Treat olives and avocados as a healthy source of fat and flavor rather than a calorie-free vegetable topping.

In the sidebar starting on page 82, you'll find healthy options for lunches at the top ten fast-food restaurants. Here are seven excellent lunch choices if you're eating at a casual dining restaurant:

Soups Are Super—and Why

Looking for a quick, delicious, nutritious meal? Look no further than a bowl of soup. Better yet, it can help you lose weight and manage your weight. A recent study found people who ate a broth-based vegetable soup before a meal consumed 20 percent fewer calories overall than those who didn't have soup. Yet they felt equally satisfied with their meals.

Broth-based soups (as opposed to cream-based soups, which tend to be high in fat) are low in energy density. That means they have few calories per serving, yet because of the high water content, they're relatively filling. Soups with lots of vegetables and beans are also high in fiber, which adds to the satiety factor, or feeling of fullness.

Soup makes an excellent AppeSizer, because it takes time to eat. However, canned soups can be high in sodium, so look for those with less than 20 percent DV (daily value) or 480 mg of sodium per serving. Check the fat content, too, and aim for soups that contain 5 or fewer grams of fat per serving. And remember, most cans of soup have two servings, so if you eat the whole can (and who doesn't?) you need to double those numbers. In short, the more vegetables and beans you have in a soup, the better.

10 second take-away:

- A bowl of soup before a meal can help you lose weight without trying.
- Opt for broth-based soups with lots of vegetables and beans for the biggest nutrient bang for your bowl.

- *Salmon salad*. Order a sautéed, 5-ounce piece of salmon and have it served on 2 cups of salad greens with a splash (2 teaspoons) of olive oil and squirt with lemon.
- *Burger & greens*. Order a 5-ounce hamburger or turkey burger with 1 slice of melted cheese, served on a bed of greens with a splash (1 to 2 tablespoons) of balsamic vinaigrette.
- *Shrimp fajitas*. Order 1 cup of grilled shrimp and mixed grilled veggies, wrapped in a flour tortilla (whole-wheat if possible).
- *Grilled chicken & veggies*. Order a 5-ounce grilled chicken breast with a 1/2 plate of grilled or steamed seasonal veggies; if you want some carbs, add 1/2 cup of steamed brown rice or a small baked potato.
- *Sushi love*. Enjoy 1 sushi roll (wrapped in brown rice if possible; avoid menu items that say "spicy" or "crunchy" or are served with sauce), 1/2 cup of steamed edamame, and 1 cup of miso soup.
- *Fish & veggies*. Order a 5-ounce piece of sautéed fish with 1/2 plate of steamed or grilled seasonal veggies, with a 1/2 cup of steamed brown rice or small baked potato.
- *Chinese delight*. Order 1/2 cup of stir-fried or steamed protein (like beef, shrimp, or chicken) with 1 cup of stir-fried or steamed mixed vegetables and 1/2 cup of steamed rice (brown, if possible) and a splash of low-sodium soy sauce.

LACKLUSTER LUNCHES:
BEATING THE EXCUSES

With all these options (even fast food), why aren't we eating a healthy lunch? I hear six major excuses—oops, I mean reasons—and once you know what they are, you'll be equipped to battle them:

I've Got No Time!

This is the number one excuse for skipping breakfast, and also the most popular reason for missing lunch. You've got no time to eat, or if you can find the time, you have no time to plan a healthy

OUR FAVORITE FAST FOOD PLACES

Hurrying through the drive-thru or running inside for a quick bite to eat? You're not alone. Americans love fast food, which may be good news for our wallets, but bad news for our waistlines. According to recent statistics, three fourths of us are trying to eat healthier when we dine out, so I'll give you a little help. Here are the ten largest quick-service restaurant chains, in order, in the United States:

- McDonald's
- Burger King
- Wendy's
- Subway
- Taco Bell

- Starbucks
- KFC (Kentucky Fried Chicken)
- Pizza Hut
- Dunkin' Donuts
- Sonic Drive-In

Even though I advise you to limit fast food, sometimes it's the only option. Below you'll find relatively healthy suggestions for the most popular fast food places, along with estimated calorie counts. Keep in mind that not all these meals and snacks fit into the ideal mix of protein and fiber, and may be higher in calories, fat, and/or sodium than what you typically want to eat. But eating right when time is tight isn't about perfection—it's about making better choices and eating a healthful balance of foods over time.

Finally, keep in mind these are possible options. Check the nutrition information in the store or online to find other good nutritional bets, as menu items often change.

McDonald's

Breakfast
Egg McMuffin (300)
Sausage Burrito (300)
Fruit 'n Yogurt Parfait (130-160 with granola)

Lunch/Dinner
Regular Hamburger (250) or Cheeseburger (300) and Small French Fries (230)
Premium Grilled Chicken Classic Sandwich (420)
Any Premium Salad with Grilled Chicken (220-320) topped with Low-Fat Dressing (40-60)
Any Snack Wrap with Grilled Chicken (260-270) and Snack Size Fruit and Walnut Salad (210)

Snacks

Fruit n' Yogurt Parfait (130-160 with granola)

Apple Dippers (35) with Low-Fat Caramel Dip (70)

Snack-Sized Fruit and Walnut Salad (210)

Burger King

Breakfast

Ham Omelet Sandwich (270)

Breakfast Burrito: Potato, Egg, Cheese and Salsa (320) or Bacon, Egg, Cheese and Salsa (300)

3 Pancakes (310) topped with 1 ounce Breakfast Syrup (70)

Lunch/Dinner

Flame-Broiled Hamburger (260) or Cheeseburger (310) and Value French Fries (220)

Tendergrill Chicken Garden Salad (230) topped with Light or Fat-Free Dressing (60-120)

BK Veggie Burger (400-450 with cheese)

Whopper JR. Sandwich (340) and Side Salad (40) topped with Light or Fat-Free Dressing (60-120)

Snacks

BK Fresh Apple Fries (25) with Caramel Sauce (45)

Garden Salad (70) topped with Light or Fat-Free Dressing (60-120)

4-piece Chicken Tenders (180)

Wendy's

Breakfast

Closed

Lunch/Dinner

Sour Cream and Chives Baked Potato (330) topped with Buttery Best Spread (50)

Large Chili (330) topped with Saltine Crackers (25) and Shredded Cheddar Cheese (70)

Jr. Hamburger (230) or Jr. Cheeseburger (270) and Kid's Meal French Fries (210)

Ultimate Chicken Grill Sandwich (340) and Side Salad (35) with Light or Fat-Free Dressing (70-90)

Mandarin Chicken Salad (180) with Roasted Almonds (130) and Crispy Noodles (70) topped with 1/2 packet of Oriental Sesame Dressing (85)

Snacks
    Small Chili (220)
    Grilled Chicken Go Wrap (250)
    Mandarin Orange Cup (90) and Low Fat Milk (100)

Subway

Breakfast
    Any Egg Muffin Melt (180-220)

Lunch/Dinner
    Any 6" Sub with 6 Grams of Fat or Less (230-380) and bowl of
    Minestrone Soup (90)

Snacks
    1 bowl of Tomato Garden Vegetable with Rotini Soup (90) and
    Apple Slices (35)
    1 packet of Raisins (130) and Light Yogurt (80)
    Any Salad with 6 Grams of Fat or Less (50-140) and Fat-Free
    Italian Dressing (35)

Taco Bell

Breakfast
    Closed

Lunch/Dinner
    Fresco Bean Burrito (340) or Fresco Burrito Supreme with
    Chicken or Steak (330-340) and side of Mexican Rice (130)
    2 Fresco Soft Tacos—Ranchero Chicken or Grilled Steak (320-
    340)
    1 Fresco Crunchy or Soft Taco (300) and side of Pintos 'n
    Cheese (170)

Snacks
    Pintos 'n Cheese (170)
    Mexican Rice (130)
    1 Fresco Crunchy or Soft Taco (150)

Starbucks

Breakfast
    Perfect Oatmeal (140) with Dried Fruit (100), Nut Medley (100)
    and Brown Sugar (50)
    Spinach, Roasted Tomato, Feta and Egg White Wrap (280)
    Reduced-Fat Turkey Bacon, Cholesterol-Free Egg White,
    Reduced-fat White Cheddar Breakfast Sandwich (340)
    Any Yogurt Parfait (290-310)
    Apple Bran Muffin with Omega-3s (350)

Lunch/Dinner

Fruit and Cheese Plate (380) or Protein Plate (370)

Chicken and Vegetable Wrap (290) and Deluxe Fruit Blend (90)

Turkey and Swiss Sandwich (390)

Snacks

Farmer's Market Salad (230)

Greek Yogurt Honey Parfait (290)

1 ounce or 24 Almonds (170)

KFC (Kentucky Fried Chicken)

Breakfast

Closed

Lunch/Dinner

Toasted Wrap with Grilled Fillet (300) and Three Bean Salad (70)

1 Skinless, Grilled Chicken Breast (190) and 1 Skinless, Grilled Drumstick (70), Green Beans (20) and Mashed Potatoes with Gravy (120)

Grilled Chicken BLT Salad (220) topped with Fat-Free Hidden Valley Ranch Dressing (35) and side of BBQ Baked Beans (200)

Snacks

Any of these sides (all under 200 calories)—Green Beans; Mashed Potatoes; Corn on the Cob; BBQ Baked Beans; Sweet Kernel Corn; Macaroni Salad; Three Bean Salad; Red Beans with Sausage and Rice; 2 Light String Cheeses; Caesar Side Salad with Light or Fat-Free Dressing; House Salad with Light or Fat-Free Dressing

Pizza Hut

Breakfast

Closed

Lunch/Dinner

2 slices of a 12" Thin 'n Crispy Pizza (360-480)

2 slices of any 12" Fit 'n Delicious Pizza (300-360)

Snacks

One slice of any 12" Fit 'n Delicious Pizza (150-180)

Side or Garden salad with Light or Fat-Free Dressing (varies by location)

Dunkin' Donuts

Breakfast
1 half of a Multigrain Bagel (195) topped with Reduced-Fat Cream Cheese (100)
Reduced-Fat Blueberry Muffin (450)
Egg and Cheese on English Muffin (320)
Egg and Cheese Wake-Up Wrap (180)

Lunch/Dinner
Turkey and Cheese Sandwich (450)
Original Chicken Wrap (240) and Chicken Noodle Soup (130)
Grilled cheese flatbread (380)

Snacks
Chicken Noodle Soup (130)
Garden Salad (180) with Fat-Free Dressing

Sonic Drive-In

Breakfast
Breakfast Burrito - Ham, Egg and Cheese (440)
Jr. Breakfast Burrito (330)

Lunch/Dinner
Jr. Burger (310) and Small French Fries (200)
Grilled Chicken Salad (250) with Light or Fat-Free Dressing (40-110) and a Fresh Banana (110)
Grilled Chicken Wrap (390) and Apple Slices (35)

Snacks
Apple Slices with Fat-Free Caramel Dipping Sauce (120)
Fresh Banana (110) and one percent Milk (100)

meal, much less shop for it. If you're eating out, you may not even have time to study the menu. You grab something, wolf it down, and attack the next thing on your to-do list.

I'm at Work ... or On the Go

Lunch is the meal most often eaten away from home. According to the National Restaurant Association, Americans consume more than *50 billion* meals in restaurants and cafeterias every year.

On a typical day, there's a 40 percent chance you'll eat at least one meal away from home. If you're employed, you probably eat lunch away at least Monday through Friday. And that's where the challenge comes in. At home you may be pressed for time, but at least you know what you're eating. In restaurants, you're at the mercy of the cook. Most restaurants stay in business by offering food that tastes good—which translates into plenty of fat, salt, sugar, and calories.

No Control over Portion Sizes

In addition to tasty food, restaurants must offer food customers can afford—and especially today, we want to get our money's worth. To attract and keep customers, restaurants serve ever-growing portions. Studies show current portion sizes of foods like hamburgers and French fries are two to five times larger than their original sizes. Another frightening study found the average cookie sold in restaurants is *700 percent* larger than the USDA's recommended serving size of half an ounce. That is one big cookie!

But we don't eyeball a typical restaurant meal and think, "Hey, a family of four could survive on the sub sandwich I just ordered!" Instead we eat what's put in front of us, which is probably far more than we actually need. Even when you make a conscious effort to cut back and eat just half perhaps, that portion can still be too much at some restaurants. Then we wonder why we're stuffed, fatigued, and seem to gain weight by the day.

I'm Eating with the Gang

If you eat at work, you're likely to eat with others—and that means you're likely to eat more. In fact, the more people you eat with, the more total calories you consume. Next chapter I'll talk more about the insidious influence your dining companions can have on how and what you eat But for now, keep in mind, that the more faces you see around the table, the more you tend to eat.

The Lunch Rush—and Practical Solutions

"Having two jobs makes it difficult to plan lunch, because I don't always know if I'll have a lunch break. I try to always eat a snack around 10:30 a.m., usually cheese and crackers or toast and peanut butter. This way, if lunch time comes late, I'm not starving and don't hit the vending machines."

—Diana, 25, child care services manager

"I sometimes have to entertain clients for lunch. I usually know where we're going and plan on what I'm going to order. I try not to look at the menu. Most restaurants will accommodate any request. That's been my experience. If I'm not entertaining, I brown-bag my lunch, which is usually chicken, brown rice, and spinach. I get my GPS to point me to the nearest 7/11 where I warm up my food."

—Enrique, 42, account executive/sales

No Options—or Few of Them

If you're eating at a fast-food restaurant or trying to assemble something together from the vending machine, you may not find healthy choices. Even if you have the luxury of eating at home (although that may not seem like a luxury to a stay-at-home mom of a rambunctious toddler), a poorly stocked refrigerator can leave you eating chips and soda and calling it lunch.

The Distraction Factor

This is a major factor for working men and women. How often do you eat at your desk, or worse yet, behind the wheel of your car? You already know distracted driving is dangerous. Well, distracted eating is just as bad for your health and weight. Whether you're reading, talking on the phone, watching television, or trying to

> 66 Making time to STOP working for a lunch break away from my desk is my biggest challenge. I keep a little note near my computer, reminding me to have a proper midday meal. 99
>
> —*Theresa, 34, community planner*

> 66 I formed better eating habits while I was pregnant with my second child. I was determined to eat healthier and not gain as much baby weight as I did during my first pregnancy. I craved anything citrus with my second pregnancy so I brought lots of fruit with me to work. I found by eating smaller, more frequent meals and snacks, I avoided eating too much of the wrong food at lunch, like pizza or Chinese food. 99
>
> —*Cassandra, 38, transportation planner*

catch up on email, eating at the same time is a bad idea. You're more likely to overeat; less likely to feel satisfied with what you ate; and more likely to experience stomach upset or heartburn. Yet we keep eating/driving, eating/working, eating/reading, eating/watching TV—eating/you-name-it.

Now that you've mastered lunch, let's take a look at the most challenging meal of all: dinner. Next chapter we'll explore why this meal is a dieter's minefield and how to successfully navigate it.

THE DINING DANGER ZONE:

Supper Strategies that Work

66 My biggest challenge with dinner is deciding what to prepare and having the ingredients on hand. I deal with that challenge by planning my week on Sunday night, including the nights we may need to eat out because of the week's hectic schedule. I usually have a few back-up options if plans change.

I have several strategies for eating healthy when dining out for dinner: I know whatever portion size I'm served will be too large, so I order small or plan to split a meal with my husband. For instance, we'll each order a salad, then split an entree. I'm careful to order salads with dressing on the side so I can control the calories on my salad. If I'm ordering a side vegetable for myself or my children, I will ask the waiter to serve steamed broccoli (no butter). If I eat the food, without it being enhanced with butter, dressing, or sauce, then I know it's the healthier option. 99

—*Kayla, 36, registered nurse and mother of 4*

While lunch presents its own set of challenges (especially lack of time and lack of healthy options), dinner and the hours afterwards are your biggest danger zone. This is when most people blow it, and it's easy to understand why. By the end of the day, if you're famished, overwhelmed, and stressed, your motivation to eat healthy has all vanished. That's why on-the-go strategies are so important.

DANGEROUS DINNERS

First, let's take a closer look at why dinner is the meal where most of us make less-than-healthy choices, overeat, or both. Think about which reasons apply to you, and which present the biggest obstacles to you eating the way you'd like to in the long run.

It's My Time!

The biggest problem for most people is the timing of dinner. This meal typically represents the end of the day—finally your opportunity to relax. You've put out fires at work, taken care of the kids, run yourself ragged all day, and now you have a chance to sit down. The last thing you want to do is count calories, carbs, and fat grams, or consider whether you're getting whole-grains, two servings of veggies, and a balanced meal. You probably just want to relax and eat—and you want something that tastes good.

Your Hunger is Out of Control

If you've had a mid-afternoon snack, hunger won't be a huge issue. But most of us don't eat enough throughout the day and end up starving by the time dinner rolls around. You know now that the longer you go between meals, the more likely you are to make poor choices or overeat—and dinner is when most people do both. This is not your fault. Your body is trying to catch up on those missed calories. Remember earlier when I talked about the importance of breakfast? Here's where you see the payoff. The more healthy calories you consume before dinner, the fewer calories you're likely to consume at dinner, and afterwards.

Lack of Time

Of course this whole book is about eating well when you're pressed for time, and the dinner hour is no exception. You may not have an extra hour to cook dinner from scratch, or maybe you're trying to get a quick bite between work and the gym. Perhaps you're grabbing something while you run errands on your way home from the office. Because so many of us work far more than the traditional forty-hour week, you may not have much cooking and eating time when you actually make it home.

Family Feeding

If you're single, dinner is one thing. If you have to feed kids or you're the primary cook for you and your partner, then dinner takes on another dimension. And that dimension means taking other people's food preferences, tastes, and schedules into consideration, which can make preparing a healthy meal all but impossible. Face it—when it comes to kids, it's got to taste good. And the more children you have, the more issues arise when it comes to feeding their hungry little faces.

Too Many Faces Around the Table

If you want to lose weight, what you're about to read may make you want to consider living like a hermit. Whether you realize it or not, your eating habits are profoundly influenced by friends, family members, and even co-workers. In fact, research shows you're more likely to overeat when you dine with other people. One classic and oft-cited study found if you dine with just one other person, you'll eat about 44 percent more food than if you dine alone. If you eat with 12 people, you'll eat 76 percent more food.

Numerous other studies over the past two decades back up this information, telling us that eating with others increases the amount of food consumed. That amount can range from one-third more to three-quarters more total calories, or even higher. In one weeklong study, researchers found the average meal eaten alone consisted of 410 calories, while the average meal consumed with others was 591 calories. In another study, researchers found people tended to eat 34 percent to 45 percent more in a social setting versus eating alone—and about 75 percent more when eating with a large group.

Why? When socializing we may unconsciously eat more without realizing it. But anthropologic reasons may also contribute to this phenomena. Think about it: tens of thousands of years ago, when eating in a group you had to make sure you got your share. Today, kids who grow up in large families may end up eating faster as adults, based on the same concept. In addition, being with family and friends—the people we're most comfortable with—may increase intake because of the comfort factor.

That Glass of Wine, or Two

When you drink alcohol, even just a glass of wine, two things are likely to happen. First, you don't compensate for the calories by cutting back on food intake, which means you consume more calories overall. And alcohol reduces inhibitions, including those related to your diet, so you may wind up eating more—especially if you've been trying to lose weight. Case in point: those fried cheese sticks you'd never look at twice can seem like the perfect light appetizer after a couple of cocktails on an empty stomach. So it's no surprise that a recent review study examining research on alcohol and food consumption found that drinking alcohol tends to increase food intake. Another interesting study found people who drank alcohol before a meal ate 16 to 25 percent more than those who didn't drink alcohol—even when the food itself was bland. And the more they drank, the more they ate, apparently due to alcohol's appetite-stimulating effects.

I'm not saying you can never drink again. But if you want to enjoy a cocktail or glass of wine, mentally count it as a substitute for dessert or the bread basket. And don't drink on an empty stomach, which exacerbates alcohol's effects. [For more on weight-smart drinking see Sidebar, Drinks with Your Diet in Mind, on page 76.]

Your Dinner Plates (Really)

If you eat dinner out, you're likely to be served portions that are way too large—say two to four times normal. As we discussed in the last chapter, restaurants stay in business by serving food that tastes good—and plenty of it. But when you eat at home, you're likely to overeat too, and for a surprising reason—the size of your dinner plates. The average sizes of plates, bowls, and glasses have gone up over the years, and average portion sizes along with them. What you think of as a dessert plate could have been a dinner plate for your grandparent—and that's not a good thing.

In addition, all kinds of hidden influences may cause you to eat more, especially at dinner. Dim lighting? Makes you eat more. Listening to fast music? Makes you eat more. Eating in front of the television? Makes you eat more. You get the idea. Even the color of your kitchen can impact your appetite, making you eat more. Warm colors like yellow, red, and orange trigger appetite more than cool colors like blues and greens, which explains why fast food restaurants are decked out in these bright, warm shades. In short, your environment may be triggering you to eat more than you need—or want.

SUPER SUPPER STRATEGIES

Feel like the deck's stacked against you? In a sense, it is. But when it comes to dinner, I have four major strategies that will help you eat right when time is tight, helping you save time and save calories, too. Each strategy takes a little effort to implement, but once they become habits you'll find that the most challenging meal of the day is anything but.

Safeguard Your Environment

You just learned how factors you barely consider can impact

what, how, and how much you eat. That's why the first supper strategy (and Master Strategy 2) is to safeguard your environment. In other words, make it as easy on yourself as possible to eat right. Some things are simple—like not keeping the cookie jar on your kitchen counter. Because here's what happens: You see the cookie jar; you think, "Cookies!" Whether you're hungry or not, you open the jar and eat a cookie. Why not keep a bowl of fresh fruit out instead?

At home, use smaller plates and bowls for meals. This one simple step takes no more time than serving food on larger plates, and you'll eat less and feel more satisfied without even trying. Eating off smaller plates means smaller portions—and if you clean your plate, you must make a conscious decision to get up for seconds. And you should have to get up. Keep the food off the kitchen table. If you can easily reach into the serving bowl for a second helping, you tend to eat more.

While eating by candlelight may be relaxing, you're also likely to eat more. Being able to see what you're consuming helps you feel more satisfied. And minimize eating while reading or watching television. Both are proven to increase caloric intake without you noticing.

Use AppeSizers

I mentioned AppeSizers in the last chapter, but it's dinner where they make a huge difference. An AppeSizer forces you to eat more slowly and takes the edge off your appetite. AppeSizers include foods with high water content to help fill your stomach without adding a lot of calories. An AppeSizer also provides a transition between the rest of your day and your evening meal, making you less likely to eat mindlessly or consume more than you want.

AppeSizers are an exception to the rule of eating right when time is tight, because they actually require more time. But taking the time to "AppeSize" your dinner is worth it in terms of your overall health, weight, and mood. Smart, simple AppeSizers include a cup of broth-based soup; fresh vegetables and several tablespoons of hummus; a small dinner salad with light dressing or dressing on the side; and even a cup of hot tea.

Limit Your Choices

When it comes to eating better, it would seem the more choices you have, the better, right? Wrong! First off, more choices mean you need more time to make a decision. Second, more choices increase the likelihood of making a less-than-healthy choice. And third, the more choices you have, the less likely you'll be satisfied with your choice after you eat it.

That's why I suggest limiting your choices for dinner, whether you eat in or out. It's as simple as deciding "I'm going to order fish tonight." Then mentally delete anything on the menu that isn't fish. Or decide in advance what you'll order, and don't even look at the menu.

Lock up Your Kitchen

I don't meant this literally, of course. But I do suggest that after dinner, and sometimes a light dessert, you consider the kitchen *closed*. If you want to lose weight, give up the evening snacking. That's when most people overeat, and on the wrong stuff (chips, cookies, ice cream, you name it). If you simply adapt the mindset of "dinner/dessert/done," you'll find you don't have to worry about choosing healthy snacks, because you're not having any.

Now that you've got the strategies in mind, here are seven super suppers for those nights you have no time to cook:

- *Cashew shrimp stir fry*. Heat ¾ cup of microwaveable brown rice and 2 cups of frozen stir-fried vegetables in the microwave. Mix with 4 ounces of pre-cooked shrimp (or any leftover grilled lean meat, fish, or poultry) and 2 tablespoons chopped cashews. Top with 1 tablespoon low-sodium soy sauce.

- *Tuna tortilla*. Mix 1 can (4 ounces, drained) water-packed light tuna with 2 tablespoons low-fat Italian dressing. Fold into a whole-grain tortilla with 2 cups of sliced vegetables (e.g., cucumbers and carrots).

- *Broccoli pot pie*. Microwave an Amy's frozen broccoli pie (or any other healthy entrée for about 400 calories) and enjoy with 1 piece seasonal fresh fruit.

- *Chicken ease*. Heat ¾ cup skinless rotisserie chicken, 1 cup cooked seasonal vegetables, and 1/2 cup of organic microwavable whole-grain rice (e.g. Seeds of Change brand), and serve.

- *Chili out*. Mix 2 cups canned turkey or vegetarian chili (organic if possible) with 1 cup frozen veggies and microwave until cooked through. Top with 2 tablespoons shredded extra-sharp cheddar cheese and, if desired, fresh parsley or cilantro to taste.

- *Green pasta-cotta*. Cook 2 ounces of whole-wheat noodles and mix with 2/3 cup of low-fat ricotta cheese, 2 cups chopped leafy greens (e.g., spinach, escarole, and Swiss chard), 1/2 cup chopped fresh herbs (e.g. chives, basil, and parsley) and minced garlic and grated lemon peel (zest) to taste (or 1 teaspoon each of the same herbs, dried).

- *Pepperoni pizza*. Top 1 serving of whole-wheat nan bread (e.g. Lavish bread) with 1/4 cup marinara sauce, 8 organic turkey pepperoni slices (choose organic as non-organic brands are loaded with artificial ingredients), 1/2 of a diced green bell pepper, and 1/3 cup part-skim mozzarella cheese. Microwave for one to two minutes, or for a crispier version, broil for three to four minutes.

THE FATTENING FOLKS IN YOUR LIFE

Take a look around you. Are your friends fat? Are members of your family overweight? What about your neighbors and co-workers? The more overweight people around you, the more likely you are to be overweight, too.

A recent study analyzed a social network of more than 12,000 people over three decades. The researchers found if food is a major part of your social life, your friends probably feel the same way—and this may mean you *and* your friends are likely to overeat on a regular basis. And if your family members tend to struggle with their weight, you may have inherited a tendency to gain weight.

Here's what researchers found regarding how the people in our lives affect our weight:

- If you have a friend who becomes obese, your chances of becoming obese increase by more than 50 percent;
- If you have a sibling who becomes obese, you are 40 percent more likely to "supersize" your body; and
- If your spouse (or partner) becomes obese, you're 37 percent more likely to become half of a chubby couple.

You may not be able to influence the eating habits of your friends and family (except for your kids), but what about your mate? Going from single status to part of a couple is likely to make you gain weight—especially if you try to keep pace with your guy. Men require more calories than women, and simply spending more time with the opposite sex can increase your intake. Not only do guys eat larger portions than women, they also tend to prefer high-fat foods (think steak, burgers, pizza, chips) that can lead to diet disasters for women.

So what can women do? Forget about trying to keep up with him forkful by forkful—it's not going to happen. Sure, you can have a pizza occasionally, but watch your portion size. Your healthy habits may affect the way he eats, but don't make it your mission in life to help him eat better. Setting a positive example may influence him, and cooking or choosing healthy meals may get him on the eat-right bandwagon. Or maybe not. You only have control over what you eat, so focus on that and let him be in charge of his own plate.

DINING OUT

How do you eat right when time is tight and you're eating out? The challenges you face depend on your typical day, so let's start with eating out at sit-down restaurants. First, consider your restaurant choices. If you have any say in the matter, suggest places where you're likely to find healthy choices. If you're stuck (say, you're eating with your boss, who insists on his favorite barbecue joint), you'll have to be more creative.

Next, try not to be starving when you sit down. Remember the study on fasting I mentioned last chapter? Bottom line, the hungrier you are, the more you'll be tempted to order high-fat, high-calorie choices—and the faster your resolve flies out the window. If you can't grab a quick snack (even a piece of fruit or a handful of nuts) on your way out the door, look for an AppeSizer food to order when you arrive.

Read the Menu

When dining at a sit-down restaurant, take a careful look at the menu before you order. I suggest you skip the entire appetizer (not to be confused with AppeSizer) section. These choices are almost always high in fat. Many restaurants offer "lite" choices that feature meals lower in fat and calories; sometimes they're designated by a special symbol on the menu. (Any doubts? Ask your server.) Next, take a look at what types of food are offered and how they're prepared. An originally healthy option (say, salmon) isn't such a great choice if it's smothered in butter. Or consider whole-grain pasta. This is an excellent entrée if you have it served with marinara sauce (and watch your portions), but when it's swimming in carbonara (a cream-based sauce with bacon and peas) or Alfredo sauce, your meal is loaded with fat.

I'm sure you already know fried foods and cream sauces are not healthy choices, but I find it's the degree of difference that often shocks people. For example, a popular sit-down restaurant serves up a whopping 1,100 calories and 61 grams of fat in its pasta carbonara entrée, while the similar-sized penne marinara entrée contains only 600 calories and 18 grams of fat.

So what do you look for? In general, limit foods that are sautéed in butter or oil. Even "salads" like potato salad and macaroni salad tend to be high in fat because they're mayonnaise-based. A chef's salad is loaded with ham, bacon, and cheese. Skip the fried foods (sorry, I can't let you count fried green beans as a vegetable), and pay attention to the way foods are described. Calling something "crispy," "crunchy," "crackling," or "batter-dipped," means it's deep-fried. You may know this already, but putting it into practice and avoiding those fat-laden choices makes a big difference.

What are smart choices? Clear, broth-based soups; lean meats, poultry or fish that is braised, broiled, grilled, or baked; and "au jus" sauces rather than gravies or cream sauces. Words like "broiled" or "stir fried" or "steamed" usually denote low-fat dishes.

Look for sides like fresh vegetables, and ask if they can be steamed or grilled instead of sautéed in butter. Ask for a plain baked potato with butter served on the side rather than mashed potatoes with cream and butter added. Request that salad dressings always be served on the side, and ask whether sauces and gravies can be left off your food.

If you've never asked questions about the way food is prepared or requested a special dish in a restaurant, you may be nervous bringing it up. Don't be. If you're polite, almost any request will be granted. Most servers are more than happy to accommodate you. If you don't have any say in how your food is prepared (say you're at a dinner party where everyone is served the same meal), simply make the best of it. Scrape off the fatty sauces, fill up on vegetables, and take a bite or two of dessert rather than deny yourself entirely. It's one thing to try to eat better, it's another for everyone to notice. No one wants to have their food choices criticized or critiqued, so don't be afraid to "go with the flow" a bit if that makes it easier for

Smart Suppers: How Real People Handle the Dinner Dilemma

Here's how four busy, health-conscious people handle dinner:

66 I'm not much of a junk food fan. I actually don't like it very much. Once a person gets used to eating vegetables, fruits, and whole grains, highly processed foods don't taste as good. So I avoid fast food places, except for Fresh Mex and perhaps a Subway, where I will have a veggie sandwich. I also avoid the big chain restaurants, such as Olive Garden, Macaroni Grill, Cheesecake Factory, etc., where the portions are large and the food is usually high in sodium, fat and calories. I trend toward vegetarian Asian, including Japanese, Thai, and Indian. I limit my portions and take food home. 99

—Sam, 53, professional writer

66 I'm fortunate to have a lot of flexibility when it comes to dinner, because it's just me. But I suppose my biggest challenge is cooking for one. I make simple things that are easy to fix, such as a wrap or snack foods I can make a meal out of. When I eat out lately, my strategy is to always look at

you. Just avoid making a bad choice and ordering food you don't want simply to appease the crowd. Standing up for yourself and your health may inspire others to do the same.

One more thing to keep in mind when dining out: portion size. As if you didn't know, they're totally out of control. And you've probably discovered that the more food you're served, the more you eat, regardless of how hungry you are. So what can you do? When the food arrives, divide it in half (or thirds, if necessary) and plan on taking the leftovers home. Have your server clear your plate as soon as you're finished, because it's easy to keep nibbling fish as my first choice since I don't fix it at home a lot and I love it. The sides offered with a fish entree are almost always steamed vegetables, which makes getting a whole healthy meal easy. 99

—Cindy, 44, employee relations specialist

66My biggest challenge when it comes to eating dinner is having the energy to make something healthy after a long day. I try to fix two or three low-fat, low-cal, heart-healthy recipes on Sunday, so during the week I only have to make a salad, which is easy, and heat up a portion of the dishes I have already made. Saves time, and also doesn't give me an excuse to get something quick. 99

—Maureen, 34, museum docent

66As a mother of three small kids my biggest challenge is finding something healthy that all three will eat. I try to have one thing I know they'll eat, and then they can have cottage cheese or peanut butter toast if they don't like the other things we're having. 99

—Angie, 35, stay-at-home mom of 3

here and there after you're no longer hungry.

Last chapter, I talked about how challenging eating out can be, and dinner is a special challenge. Your day is almost over, you want to unwind and relax, and you're more likely to drink alcohol than at any other meal. Plus, you typically spend more time at dinner than any other meal, which is a good thing to help you "eat aware" (Master Strategy 4) and spend at least twenty minutes eating a meal. But the key is to take the portion you want and then get the rest out of sight, because the longer you sit at the table with food in front of you, the more you eat.

Now that you've got a handle on the "three squares," let's move on to the other element of eating right on the go: smart snacking. In the next chapter you'll learn why you need to snack, how to snack smart, and how eating more frequently can not only make you feel better and give you more energy, but result in lasting weight loss.

6

SUPERCHARGE YOUR SNACKS:

Eat More Frequently, Lose Weight

66 I do snack during the day. I like baby carrots, celery, an apple with peanut butter or a banana. My standard go-to is light flavored yogurt. I've recently tried the "dessert" flavors (red velvet cake, key lime pie) that help satisfy a sweet tooth. Sometimes it is cheese and crackers, salsa and chips, or popcorn. On some days I go for mini candy bars and devour five, or chips and dip, but those days are few compared to when I choose healthy options. I do believe choosing the healthy, fresh snacks helps me maintain my weight because they're not processed, not loaded with sodium and saturated fat, and they keep me feeling full longer than snacks filled with empty calories. 99

—*Jill, 28, corporate communications writer*

When it comes to snacking, the question isn't *whether* you've snacked today, but *what* snacks you ate. New research shows we've become a nation of snackers. A whopping 97 percent of Americans

Are All Waters Created Equal?

Reach for a bottle of water these days and you may be wondering which one to pick. Enhanced waters first came on the scene when researchers started developing waters for athletes training and competing at high levels. The first beverages contained electrolytes and/or carbohydrates, but they were just the beginning. Now we can choose from a variety of "designer" waters, and you may be amazed at what they include.

Some enhanced waters contain additional vitamins and minerals; others contain caffeine, guarana, and other stimulants; others have fiber, and herbs like ginseng. While their labels may make impressive claims (like "restore and bring balance to your body" or "hydrate and replenish the body with essential vitamins and minerals"), don't get too excited. The effect of these beverages isn't well-studied and it's doubtful waters containing extra vitamins, minerals, or anything else will make a major difference in your health or your day. If you're a serious athlete, and exercise for more than an hour at a time, then electrolyte-enhanced beverages may improve your performance. But for most of us, it's just water with extra stuff—and added calories.

However, some people find flavored water more palatable, so if these designer beverages appeal to you, give them a try. Just choose ones that have no added sugar or artificial flavors. Even if they contain vitamins or other "bonus ingredients," don't expect miracles.

10 second take-away:

- Aim to drink at least six to eight 8-ounce glasses of water a day for optimal hydration.
- Choose enhanced waters if you like the taste, but look for ones with no added sugar or artificial flavoring. If you're a serious athlete, electrolyte-enhanced beverages may help your performance.

snack daily (up from 71 percent thirty years ago). If you're any-thing like the average person, snacks now contribute one-quarter of calories to your daily intake. On average, they comprise 579 calories (up from 357 calories, or 14 percent of daily intake, thirty years ago). So it's easy to see why experts are blaming fat- and sugar-laden snacks (think potato chips, soda, candy, fruit drinks, and even "energy" bars) for our ever-expanding waistlines.

But snack is not a four-letter word. (It's actually five letters—but you get the point.) Yes, when it comes to eating healthy or losing weight, people think of snacks as bad. And yes, a giant bag of fried

Get the Most Energy from Your Energy Bar

If you're on the go, an energy bar may seem like a smart snack. But with literally dozens of brands to choose from in a variety of flavors, which do you choose? Is a granola-based bar better than a protein bar? Should you grab a bar that promises a 40/30/30 blend of carbs, protein, and fat? Do you need a bar made especially for women?

Here's the thing: some energy bars are a great nutritional deal. But many of these attractively packaged bars are little more than vitamin-fortified candy, with calories and taste coming from high fructose corn syrup and other forms of sugar. Your best bet is to look for bars with "whole" ingredients (whole soy, fruit, and nuts, for example) that clock in at 200 calories or less.

Bars containing fruit may be relatively high in sugar, but to limit added sugar, choose bars that contain 18 grams or less of sugar per serving. And look for bars with at least 3 grams of fiber and 4 grams of protein to help meet Master Strategy 1.

10 second take-away:
- Choose energy bars with "whole" food ingredients—you should recognize what you're eating.
- Select bars that contain 200 calories or fewer, and less than 18 grams of sugar.

Overcoming Cravings

In a chapter about snacking, I'd be remiss if I didn't talk about cravings. One survey of college students found 97 percent of women and 68 percent of men experienced food cravings, defined as "a strong desire to eat a particular food." On average, the students experienced five to nine cravings a month. Women were most likely to crave chocolate, followed by salty foods, pizza, ice cream, and other sweets. Men, on the other hand, were more likely to crave pizza, followed by chocolate, meat and chicken, and sweets.

While both sexes experience food cravings, women are more likely to have them than men. The reason may have to do with brain chemistry—women are more sensitive to changes in blood sugar levels than men, so when blood sugar levels drop they're more likely to crave high-sugar foods. Women also produce less serotonin, a brain chemical that improves mood. Lack of serotonin may explain why women are more susceptible to conditions like depression and seasonal affective disorder than men. Craving starchy carbs like bread and pasta may be your body's way of trying to self-medicate and produce more serotonin.

Hormonal changes also play a role in food craving. Women experience more food cravings premenstrually, during perimenopause, and after giving birth. During all three of those times, estrogen levels drop, which causes a corresponding drop in brain serotonin. Premenstrual food cravings may also be the result of your body needing more calories, because your metabolism revs up slightly in the days before your period begins.

But food cravings often have an even simpler explanation. If you've been trying to lose weight and slashed your caloric intake too drastically, you're more likely to desire high-calorie, high-fat foods. Your body is reminding you it needs fuel to function. When you don't eat enough, you'll probably be plagued with food cravings until you give in.

Eliminating all fat from your diet can also backfire. Fat is a necessary nutrient and helps you feel full after eating; it also releases endorphins in your brain which have a mood-enhancing effect. Another brain chemical called galanin is elevated in the afternoon and stimulates fat cravings. If you eat a little fat, your galanin will drop back to normal, but if you ignore it, the craving for high-fat food may get worse.

So what can you do? If you're experiencing a craving, distinguish whether it's physical or emotional in nature. Are you truly hungry? Or do you just want to make yourself feel better, or distract yourself, with the food you're thinking of? A big glass of water and a healthy snack will often take the edge off your craving.

To experience fewer cravings, fuel your body every three to five hours (Master Strategy 8). Regular workouts can also help. Exercise increases levels of both serotonin—a lack of which can trigger carbohydrate cravings—and endorphins—a lack of which can produce fat cravings. People who work out frequently report reduced food cravings.

But hey, sometimes you just crave something sweet. If that's the case, here are seven simple, smart snacks that honor your sweet tooth and your waistline:

- **Nuts & chocolate**. Have 1 small handful (1/2 ounce) of nuts with 1 tablespoon of dark chocolate chips.

- **Frozen fruit bar**. Have 1 frozen 100 percent fruit bar and 1/4 cup of reduced-fat ricotta cheese with a drizzle of honey on top.

- **Greek yogurt & jam**. Mix 1/2 cup of plain low-fat Greek yogurt with 1 tablespoon of 100 percent fruit spread or jam of choice.

- **Hot cocoa**. Make 1 cup of hot chocolate with low-fat or nonfat milk.

- **Ricotta & fruit.** Top 1 slice of melon with 1/4 cup of reduced-fat ricotta cheese and a pinch of cinnamon or cardamom, and enjoy with one full-sheet graham cracker.

- **Strawberries-n-cream**. Mix 1 cup plain low-fat Greek yogurt with a drizzle each of honey and balsamic vinegar, and serve as a dip with 1 cup of fresh strawberries on stems.

- **Sorbet**. Have 1/2 cup of sorbet of your choice with a few (about 10) chopped nuts.

tortilla chips or a gooey chocolate bar is a poor choice. But if you change the way you approach snacks and start thinking of them not as junk food, but as mini-meals, something wonderful happens. You improve your nutrient intake, maintain your energy level, and lose weight.

I often tell clients they can snack themselves thin. Snacking is simply the natural extension of "energize in 3-5," (Master Strategy 8) or eat every three to five hours. Feeding your body at regular intervals actually helps you lose weight, because you maintain consistent blood sugar levels and never become ravenous. Choose smart snacks and you'll also wind up boosting your overall fruit and vegetable intake.

Making Snacks Work

Hey, 97 percent of us snack, and snacks can be healthy, remember? Here's how two real people make snacks work for them:

66 Eating small snacks more often prevents me from binging, because I never reach that "CRAZY" point. 99

Nicole, 38, attorney

66 I do snack during the day. My downfall is that if it's in the house, I'll probably be attracted to eating it. My husband and I are on the same page nutritionally. That's very important, because I don't feel like I have to grocery shop for everyone's taste. I purchase fast snacks that are healthy (mini carrots, apples, bananas, etc.) Holidays are hard because we end up with more high-calorie/less-nutritious foods in the house. I have learned to throw food in the garbage without feeling guilty—if there's too much Halloween candy left over, I throw it out. 99

Kayla, 36, registered nurse, mother of 4

I'm not the only one who believes snacking is good for you. Recent research tells us that smart snacking can make you feel better and enhance your performance at work and at home:

- One study found that dividing calories into four smaller meals over six hours, instead of having two larger meals, improved participants' verbal reasoning.
- A study that examined the eating patterns of almost 16,000 U.S. adults found those who ate three meals and two or more snacks a day had the highest levels of nutrients including folic acid, vitamin C, calcium, magnesium, potassium, and fiber than those who ate fewer snacks.
- A study of wildland firefighters found those who consumed an eat-on-move ration (in other words, a portable snack) were able to work harder—in essence, do more firefighting work—than those who didn't have the portable snack.
- Another study found that children who had a mid-morning snack were able to concentrate better on schoolwork than kids who did not.

Here's the thing—if you want to lose weight, you might think the fewer calories a snack has, the better. Not true. While a handful of carrot sticks may take the edge off your hunger, they won't keep you going for long. Snacks that include a combination of fiber and protein (Master Strategy 1) give you sustained energy for hours. So instead of having a piece of fruit or a half a whole-grain bagel (both of which contain some fiber but no protein), put a little peanut butter on your apple slices, or add turkey or a slice of cheese to your bagel.

Another bonus is that eating well throughout the day can stave off the nighttime munchies. If you take in too few calories during the day, you may be so hungry by the time you get home that you'll wind up polishing off hundreds of extra calories. And here's something you may not have thought of: taking the time to eat a healthy snack forces you to take a break during a nutty, crazed day. I realize you may gobble your snack behind the wheel or sneak bites during a meeting, and that's understandable. But if you can take just five minutes to eat your snack without multi-tasking, you'll also give yourself a brief reprieve that may help your mood and reduce your overall stress.

Taking the time to work out *gives* you time (in terms of increased energy, better mood, and overall improved productivity). Taking the time to snack will also give you time.

I want to clarify one point. Smart snacking doesn't mean mindless eating, or grabbing whatever you can find. Most people I work with fall into two basic categories. The first are people too

Too Much Sweet Stuff: The Skinny on Added Sugar

How much sugar do you consume? Chances are it's more than you think—and that can be bad for your overall health and weight. The American Heart Association (AHA) recently issued specific guidelines limiting sugar consumption. Too much sugar isn't just bad for your teeth—it makes you more likely to gain weight and can affect your heart health as well. That's why the AHA says most women should consume 100 calories a day (or less) of added sugar, and men 150 calories or less. That's not a lot—about 6 teaspoons of added sugar for women, and 9 for men.

Yet most Americans consume about 22 teaspoons (355 calories' worth) of added sugar a day. A major source of sugar for many of us is found in sodas, which may contain up to 10 teaspoons of added sugar in one 12-ounce can.

Check the package to help determine how much added sugar a food has. Some packages will say "sugar-free" or "contains no added sugar." Read the ingredient list; the higher up you find sugar, the more sugar the product has. And remember you're not just looking for the word "sugar." Ingredients like cane juice, cane syrup, corn sweetener, corn syrup, dextrose, high fructose corn syrup, and sucrose all mean "sugar."

busy to snack. I must talk them into it. Yet they find that taking a few extra minutes to fit healthy snacks into their day (especially the afternoon) makes a big difference in how they eat and feel.

Now let's talk about the second kind. These are people who snack too much, too often, or both. If this sounds like you, chances are you're snacking for reasons other than hunger. Maybe you use a snack as a reward for getting something done, as a distraction, or simply because it tastes good. There's nothing wrong with that once in a while, but if you're in the habit of snacking on whatever's handy regardless of whether you're hungry, you'll set yourself up for a weight problem (if you don't have one already).

If you're a constant muncher, before you snack I suggest you

The Nutrition Facts label tells how much sugar a food has per serving, but doesn't distinguish between added sugar and naturally occurring sugar. Watch for high fructose corn syrup and avoid it when you can. High fructose corn syrup is generally found in cheap, processed food and your body may turn it to fat faster than other types of sugar. Limiting it as much as possible will also help you cut unnecessary sugar, as it is "hidden" in so many foods.

Simply cutting back your consumption of non-diet sodas, juice (even 100 percent fruit juice is high in naturally-occurring sugar), candy, sweetened cereals, and baked goods (cookies, doughnuts, and pastries) will help limit your sugar intake. Look for fruit packed in its own juice or in water rather than syrup. And if you crave something sweet, reach for the fruit first—grapes, a banana, or strawberries may take the edge off your sugar craving.

10 second take-away:
- Cut back on sodas, candy, juice, and baked goods to reduce your hidden sugar intake.
- Read labels and avoid high fructose corn syrup whenever you can.

"check in" with your body and make sure you're truly physically hungry. If you're really hungry, even a healthy snack will sound delicious. If you're just eating to eat, it's not about satisfying your hunger, it's about just eating something. [See Sidebar, Overcoming Cravings, for more on distinguishing between physical and emotional hunger, on page 108.]

If you're in the habit of snacking all the time, you'll find eating specific snacks will help you break the habit of just eating whatever, whenever. And healthy snacks *can* taste good and be satisfying. The key is choosing ones you like and watching your portions. Here are seven snacks to keep on hand at home or in your office fridge:

Go Nuts—Really!

Nuts sometimes get a bad rap for being high in calories and fat, but they make an excellent snack choice. The fat in nuts is healthy fat that promotes heart health, and as long as you use portion control, the protein and fiber a handful of nuts contain can keep hunger at bay for hours.

Not all nuts are created equal, however. Your best bets for nutrition are almonds, walnuts, and pistachios. Almonds are the richest in vitamin E; walnuts contain a plant-based omega-3 fatty acid; and pistachios have lutein and zeaxanthin, carotenoids important for eye health. Research shows nut eaters are generally thinner, less likely to develop type 2 diabetes, and have a reduced risk of developing cardiovascular disease. Here's what a one-ounce serving of nuts actually looks like and how many calories each contains:

- Almonds: 23 almonds = 160 calories
- Cashews: 18 cashews = 160 calories
- Hazelnuts: 21 hazelnuts = 180 calories
- Macadamias: 10-12 macadamias = 200 calories
- Pecans: 19 halves = 200 calories
- Pistachios: 49 pistachios = 160 calories
- Walnuts: 14 halves = 190 calories

- *Hummus lovin'.* Spread 2 tablespoons of hummus on a 1/2 warmed whole-wheat pita, or serve the hummus with a 1/2 pint of cherry tomatoes.
- *Fruit & cheese.* Have 1 ounce of cheese with 1 fresh pear or 1 cup of grapes.
- *Yogurt & fruit.* Serve 1 cup of nonfat, plain Greek yogurt with a 1/2 cup of seasonal fresh fruit and a drizzle of honey.
- *Edamame.* Have 1 cup of steamed, whole edamame sprinkled with a pinch of coarse sea salt.
- *Fruit & nut butter.* Have 1 small, crisp apple with 1 tablespoon of all-natural nut butter.

Nut butters (hey, peanut butter is just the beginning) are another way to boost protein and fiber intake, but some are high in added sugars. Choose all-natural nut butters with as few ingredients as possible. For example, I usually choose an almond butter jar that contains "dry roasted almonds" as its ingredients list—that's it! Some may also contain sea salt.

10 second take-away:
- Stash single-servings of nuts for a quick, portion-controlled snack.
- Choose an all-natural nut butter that contains just one or two ingredients (e.g., dry roasted cashews and sea salt).

- *Cottage cheese please*. Serve 1 cup of low-fat cottage cheese with a 1/2 cup of seasonal fresh fruit or veggies—or with 5 brown rice or other whole-grain crackers.
- *Turkey roll-ups*. Spread 3 turkey slices with Dijon mustard, add mixed baby greens (and thinly sliced onion if desired), and roll them up before eating.

Of course you may not be near a refrigerator, so here are seven easy snacks you can pick up at a convenience store or gas station:

Eat "Green" on the Go: Keeping Planet Earth in Mind

The biggest move in eating right these days is eating green. And that doesn't just mean eating more green leafy vegetables—it means eating with an eye toward sustainability and maintaining the earth's limited natural resources.

Eating on the run and eating to help the earth aren't mutually exclusive. Here are seven ways you can eat green without slackening the pace of your life:

- Buy the largest size packaging of foods, and portion your own servings to control your servings and create less waste. (You'll save money, too.)
- Choose reusable containers for snacks and on-the-go meals.
- Invest in a reusable water bottle and fill it at home or work, saving hundreds (maybe thousands) of dollars on bottled water, not to mention the hassle of buying plastic bottles.
- Buy local when you can. The shorter distance food has to travel to reach you, the fewer resources are used to transport it.
- Recycle whenever you can. Most communities offer curbside pickup now.
- When you have more than one choice, select the product with less packaging.
- Buy organic foods when you can. [See Sidebar, The Big O, on page 70.]

- **Seeds please**. Have 1 ounce (a handful) roasted sunflower or pumpkin seeds.
- **Egg it**. Have 1 hard-boiled egg and 1 small container of low-sodium vegetable juice.
- **Bar it**. Have 1 whole-food bar. [See Sidebar, Get the Most Energy from Your Energy Bar, on page 107.]
- **Apple & cheese**. Have 1 package of apple slices or 1 ounce of dried fruit with 1 piece of string cheese. (Choose dried fruit without the preservative sulphur dioxide, which may be harmful for people with allergies, and children, especially those with asthma or food intolerances.)
- **Soy chips**. Have 1 single-serve bag of soy chips, which provide protein and fiber.
- **Shell it**. Have 1 ounce of pistachios (49 nuts).
- **Yogurt & fruit**. Have 1 cup low-fat yogurt with a fruit leather (a strip of dried fruit).

WATER WORKS: ARE YOU GETTING ENOUGH H2O?

Now you know that snacking can improve your performance and mood throughout the day. Yet there's another factor to satiety and performance that most of us never think about.

Let me ask you this: what did you eat yesterday? You can probably answer that question fairly easily. But what if I ask how much, and what fluids, you drank? Unless you're a serious athlete, chances are you've downplayed the importance of hydration.

Most people don't realize that water is actually considered one of the six classes of nutrients. Water is critical to good health, especially if you want to lose weight or maintain a healthy weight, because your body needs a certain amount of water to function properly. You're 60 percent water by weight, and water is used for everything from converting food into energy to carrying nutrients and oxygen to regulating your temperature.

Yet you may be walking around chronically dehydrated—and

it's not your fault. If you only drink when you feel thirsty, you're probably not drinking enough. Your body's thirst mechanism kicks in relatively slowly. By the time you're thirsty, you're already 2 percent dehydrated, enough to impact your mood and energy level.

Chances are you drink less than the oft-heard recommendation "eight 8-ounce glasses" of water a day. Just keep in mind that this commonly cited rule is only an estimate. Your personal hydration needs may be less, or more, than that amount, depending on your

Pack Your Eat Right Survival Stash

You're stuck in traffic and starving, but you have no food in the car. Your boss just called an emergency meeting and you'll have nothing to eat except the platter full of giant cookies everyone else is munching on. Or you just had a terrible day and want something sweet to soothe your chocolate craving—without totally blowing your healthy eating plans. That's where an ER (Eat Right) Survival Stash comes in handy. It's your emergency plan when the unexpected happens.

I suggest you keep an ER Survival Stash in the following locations:
- Your office/workplace;
- Your car;
- Your purse or briefcase; and
- Your suitcase or carry-on bag.

What will your ER Survival Stash contain? That's up to you, but here are four suggestions for satisfying, healthy snacks on the go:
- *Go nuts*. A 200-calorie "snack pack" of nuts (buy pre-portioned bags or make your own).
- *Bar it*. A whole-food bar [See Sidebar , Get the Most Energy from Your Energy Bar, on page 107].
- *Veg out*. 1 ounce (1/4 cup) of dried veggies and a small handful (1/2 ounce) of soy nuts for protein.
- *Fruit up*. 1 ounce (1/4 cup) of preservative-free dried fruit with a small handful (1/2 ounce) of nuts for protein.

body weight, your activity level, the season of the year, and your diet. Up to about 20 percent of your body's water needs can come from food, especially fruits and vegetables that are naturally high in water.

Drinking more water isn't just good for your health. Water may help you lose weight, too. One study found overweight women who increased their water intake from less than one liter (or about four 8-ounce glasses) per day to more than one liter per day lost nearly 5 pounds over the course of the year—without changing anything else about their lifestyles. And thirst often masquerades as hunger, so drinking water or a beverage like unsweetened tea can take the edge off your appetite—and help you naturally eat less over time.

So how do you know you're short on water? You may have trouble concentrating, feel tired, or wind up eating more than usual. As I just mentioned, it's common to misinterpret thirst as hunger. Other symptoms of dehydration include lightheadedness, headache, loss of appetite, flushed skin, and dry mouth and eyes. And one of the easiest ways to track hydration is by checking your urine. Sounds weird, but it's true. If your pee is plentiful and straw-colored, you're drinking enough. If it's scanty or dark yellow, you need to boost your fluid intake. (Just keep in mind that some dietary supplements and medications can also change the color of your urine.)

While water is always a good bet, you needn't rely only on H_2O to satisfy your fluid needs. Beverages like tea, coffee, and juice all contribute to your daily total, as do foods like soup, fruits, and vegetables that are naturally high in water content. You can up your intake by having a big glass of water first thing in the morning; keeping a bottle of water on your desk at work; drinking a glass at mid-morning and mid-afternoon; and being sure to drink before, during, and after exercise.

Now that you've learned how to snack smart and snack yourself skinny, you've got the basics of eating right when time is tight. For day-to-day life, you're all set with dozens of ideas for breakfast, lunch, dinner, and snacks. Once you get into your new routine, it will become a healthy habit that's easy to maintain.

But life likes to throw curve balls. That's why in the next chapter you'll learn how to handle anything that gets tossed your way. Vacation? Travel? Weddings? Parties? Holidays? You'll learn how to eat smart at any location and any occasion, and keep those curve balls from striking out your healthy routine.

ANYTHING BUT ROUTINE:

Special Strategies for Special Occasions

"Trying to find something healthy in airports is next to impossible. I bring along snacks I know are healthy—usually fruit, already cut up and in a Tupperware case, or sandwiches, granola bars, etc.

During the holidays I try to expand my workouts, hopefully soaking up the extra calories taken in. I know this isn't all that creative, but it's how I try to handle it. I also find if I picture the party I'm going to attend and decide I'll only have two glasses of wine, eat a half of a plate's worth of appetizers, etc., then I can follow my plan. I try to make decisions ahead of time. True, it doesn't always work, but often it does."

Maureen, 34, museum docent

Once you establish the habit of eating right on the run, smart and nutritious choices come more easily. What we eat, when, why, and how, are all dictated primarily by habit, after all. Creating a new habit takes time and effort—typically at least 21 days. But once that behavior is in place, you slip into a whole new (and hopefully healthier) groove. You've already made the decision to change your behavior, and you do so automatically and unconsciously. That's a habit.

However, while many of your days may be routine and you can act out of habit, other days will not. What happens when you have to travel for business or take a long-awaited vacation? What about attending a wedding, class reunion, or big party? And what about the number one derailer of diet intentions: the holidays?

Anything out of your ordinary routine is likely to present a

Navigating the Room Service Menu

Room service. The very phrase evokes images of enormous portions, mouth-watering food, and a variety of delicious meals, delivered to your doorstep with no effort on your part. Be careful! Almost all meals in the room service menu are high in fat and calories, and after a long day they all sound delicious.

What can you do? First, look for healthy choices. Most hotels offer at least a few items that are lower in calories and fat, often denoted with a special symbol. Otherwise, make the best choice you can, choosing a meal that contains protein and fiber (Master Strategy 1) and look for ways to cut back on fat. That may mean asking that a meal be served without sauce, or your vegetables be steamed rather than sautéed in butter. If you order a chef's salad, you can always ask for it without ham or bacon, or simply remove the fatty meats (and part of the cheese) before you eat.

For meal ideas, refer to the lunch and dinner choices listed in Chapters 4 and 5. And if you hit your hotel room famished, have something from your ER Survival Stash to take the edge off your appetite, or order an AppeSizer and eat it slowly before you dig into dinner.

challenge. In this chapter I'm going to help arm you with strategies to use while traveling, entertaining, vacationing, and partying—any time your usual habits are thrown out of whack.

ON THE ROAD: HANDLING BUSINESS TRAVEL

The average person spends more than three hours behind the wheel of her car every day, totaling more than twenty hours each week. If you travel frequently—or even occasionally—that means more time in planes, trains, and automobiles. And that often means throwing a massive monkey wrench into your healthy eating routine.

What's so challenging about travel? Almost everything. First, your time is not your own. Your flight is delayed, and you're stuck in the airport an extra four hours, or longer. Worse yet, you're stuck in the plane on the tarmac, waiting hours for the okay to take off. Even if you wind up driving, you can't control traffic conditions. A trip that was supposed to take you less than an hour may wind up taking three times longer, thanks to construction, traffic jams, or just plain bad luck.

Once you arrive at the destination, you may put in extra hours at the office, entertain clients late into the night, or have to prep for important presentations and meetings. At the hotel you may have to face down the mini-bar or an all-you-can eat breakfast buffet the next morning. Between stress, fatigue, overload, and jet lag, it's not surprising your energy and motivation are sapped.

That's the bad news about traveling for work. The good news? Hopefully, travel will help you keep your job. Seriously, the real good news is that you can ferret out healthy choices on the road. You've already collected advice from the preceding chapters on smart choices, so let's focus on the big challenges of business travel:

The 18-hour day. Traveling for work? As I mentioned, your time is not your own. There's no typical day when it comes to business travel—and that lack of control means you must come prepared.

Carrying your ER Survival Stash (healthy, already-portioned, shelf-stable foods) in your briefcase or bag and a bottle of water or tea is your first weapon of choice. If you're dining out alone or with clients, use the lunch and dinner strategies and meal suggestions from earlier chapters. When they've become habits, you'll spend less time deciding (or worrying about) what to eat and more time focusing on your work—which is why you're there.

Keeping up with clients. In some cases your time is limited to work, but if you entertain clients or spend time socializing with people for work, you face another hurdle. Whether attending a conference or on the road for your job, don't fall into the trap of thinking this is a free-for-all. (More about that dangerous mindset

The Breakfast Bar—What to Order

Breakfast buffets have become standard fare in most hotels. At some you may be able to order a cooked-to-order omelet, while at others the choice is limited to juice, rolls, cereal, and coffee. Here's how to make the most of the breakfast bar without getting the excess calories and fat:

- *Go easy on the juice*. Use a small glass for fruit juice, which is loaded with calories and naturally-occurring sugar. Vegetable juices like tomato are lower in calories, but high in salt.
- *Look for a high-fiber breakfast cereal*. If the choices are relatively slim, a low-sugar cereal with at least 3 grams of fiber per serving with skim or one percent milk and a piece of fresh fruit like a banana make a healthy, satisfying breakfast. Regular Cheerios (not the sugar-added varieties) is a good option and available at most breakfast buffets. Better yet, go for a hot cereal like oatmeal.
- *Maximize your options*. If the restaurant has an omelet station, ask that it be loaded up with veggies like mushrooms, onions, and spinach and go easy on, or skip, the cheese and meat. You'll start your day with a serving or two of vegetables (high in fiber and nutrients), plus protein from the eggs. Many people

in a bit.) If your job requires you to spend time with people—say, drinking, eating, and entertaining—watch what you drink, and swap mineral water with a slice of lime or lemon for alcoholic beverages. Eat a healthy dinner or use a snack from your ER Survival Stash to take the edge off your appetite. Focus on the people, not the food and drink.

Home (or rather, hotel room) at last. Finally, you've arrived at the hotel. You slip off your shoes, hang up your clothes, and sprawl on the bed. If you haven't had a chance to eat, it's room service, the mini bar, or the vending machine down the hall. If your day has been long and stressful and tiring, it's natural to want to treat yourself—or just order whatever sounds good and veg out in front

think egg whites are better, but egg yolks contain nutrients you miss out on when you limit yourself to egg whites. Another option when ordering an omelet is to request one full egg, and egg whites for the rest.

- *Skip the breads and bagels*. You'll find few whole grains at breakfast bars, so pass on the bagels, white toast, croissants, doughnuts, and other sweet breads altogether. They're high in calories, low in fiber, and may set you up for a blood sugar crash later in the morning.
- *Stock up for later*. Slip portable fruit like a banana, an apple, and a box of high-fiber cereal into your bag or briefcase to fill out your ER Survival Stash for later if you have no other food on hand.
- *Just say no ... to bacon and sausage*. Sure it may smell delicious, but it's all too easy to go overboard on these fat-laden, salty meats. Skip them altogether, or allow yourself one piece and savor it.
- *Look for ways to "veg out and fruit up."* (Master Strategy 5) at the breakfast bar. It's easier to find fruit than vegetables at breakfast, but a bowl of seasonal fresh fruit like melon or strawberries will provide plenty of fiber and vitamins to start off your morning.

of the tube or your laptop for awhile.

Whether you're staying at a three-star hotel or a chain hotel, when you first check in have a quick peek at the fitness center. Then you'll know exactly where it's located, giving you no excuse to avoid exercising first thing. If it's not too late, and depending where you're staying, look for a local market to stock up on healthy snacks—bottled water, energy bars, fresh or dried fruit, nuts, and yogurt if you have a refrigerator. Keep your ER Survival Stash on hand. Many hotels offer mini-markets where you can find many of these foods.

Make it a priority to do a quick workout first thing in the morning. Even thirty minutes on the treadmill or a twenty-minute session of lifting weights will translate into higher productivity and less stress throughout a busy day, which translates into more time. If you hate to work out, even better—you start your day by tackling and overcoming something that's a challenge for you. Great job.

The All-You-Can Eat Buffet

Personally, I find all-you-can-eat buffets scary. Most people don't need extra encouragement to eat more, and many of the dishes on the buffet are high in calories and fat. To navigate the buffet, keep these tips in mind:

- *Check out your options*. Don't just grab a plate and start loading it. Take a walk down the buffet and see what looks most appealing to you. Then get in line, and fill your plate with two healthy options and, if you need it, one portion-controlled "gotta have." Although variety is good sometimes, it spells diet disaster at the buffet table.
- *Go natural*. In other words, the more recognizable something is and the less it's had added to it, the better. Starting with the salad section of the buffet, opt for fresh vegetables and fruit, but skip the mayonnaise-laden choices like potato salad and macaroni salad.

PERSONAL TIME: VACATIONS AND OTHER TRAVEL

With business travel, you're away from home because you *have* to be. Going on vacation is a whole different thing—except you still face the lack of control (delayed flights, lost luggage, traffic hassles). Here's the biggest issue with vacations: people go overboard because they *can*. They say, "I deserve this. I've worked so hard this year. A few desserts won't kill me." [Insert your excuse of choice.] That's why many people return from vacation 4, 7, or even 10 pounds heavier. Sure, you had a fantastic time, but do you really want to be unable to zip your pants in a week?

That's why the first order of business is to let go of the "gotta-have-it" mindset. I'm not saying you can't indulge or splurge. That's part of being on vacation. But if you limit yourself even a little (you know, like having one dessert a day—not two, or even three) you'll

- *Veg out and fruit up*. It's a Master Strategy for a reason. Cover half your plate with vegetables and a little fruit and you'll eat well and leave less room for higher-calorie selections.
- *Slow down*. Take time to enjoy the food you've chosen, and don't go back for seconds just to get your money's worth.
- *Skip the breads*. As with breakfast buffets, most all-you-can-eat buffets offer a ton of refined breads and rolls. Unless you're craving bread, skip it and opt for foods higher in fiber and nutrients.
- *Make the most of the buffet*. By this, I don't mean eat as much as possible. I mean try something new if it appeals to you. You can always get fresh shrimp or grilled chicken, but if a soup or dish looks delicious, give it a try. No one expects you to forgo all pleasure, especially on vacation.
- *Finally, remember to check your portion size* (see Sidebar, Portion Patrol, on page 64). It's all too easy to overeat when waiters keep bringing new plates, which makes it's difficult to get a handle on how much you've actually eaten.

eat better and feel better too. Waking up in the morning feeling stuffed, bloated, and uncomfortable is not how you want to spend your precious vacation time.

A little balance will go a long way. I suggest you work out first thing in the morning when you're traveling for work—and traveling for pleasure as well. No, you don't have to stumble out of bed for a sunrise power yoga class. But a regular workout routine will keep some of those vacation treats from settling around your waistline.

What else can you do? Stock up on healthy snacks to have on hand as an ER Survival Stash in your hotel room—and plan to eat a meal (say breakfast) in your room most days. If you'll be on the go all day, take snacks with you, and make sure you stay hydrated. Remember that thirst often masquerades as hunger, and opt for no-calorie or low-calorie beverages throughout the day. Watch your alcohol intake—those calories add up fast, especially if you start drinking before evening—and look for ways to get more fruits and vegetables into your day.

The guidelines for eating smart on vacation are the same you would follow every day—with a bit of leeway. Eating every three to five hours (Master Strategy 9), combining protein and fiber (Master Strategy 1), getting plenty of produce (Master Strategy 5), exercising thirty minutes or more a day (Master Strategy 8), and staying hydrated (Master Strategy 7) will all help you make the most of your vacation time, without feeling like you're suffering or missing out.

FAMILIES, FETES, AND FESTIVITIES: HOLIDAYS, PARTIES, AND OTHER SOCIAL OCCASIONS

We've covered travel, whether for work or play. Now let's talk about all those social events that tend to derail your eating plan. We're talking holidays, wedding receptions, parties, even funerals. They all have something in common: they involve food, typically lots of it, mostly loaded with fat and calories.

Let's talk about social events first, and then I'll tackle holidays, which are the most challenging time of the year to cat well. (And really, the holidays are often one long list of social events.) In most cultures, socializing and food go hand-in-hand. Even when you make smart choices for meals and snacks, you're likely to overindulge, and over-imbibe, at parties and other social events.

Choose wisely. Okay, you've arrived at your neighbor's open house or the office holiday bash. The food looks delicious and smells even better. Hold on. Just as I suggested at a buffet, before you grab your plate, get an idea of what's being offered and make a plan. You may choose to skip the foods you can get anytime — crackers and cheese, say — and choose small portions of foods that are a real treat. Or you may choose to load up on fresh vegetables and fruit, if available, to fill your plate and your stomach, and take the edge off your appetite.

Stay away—from the buffet. Don't stand around the table — get what you want and move away from the food. And don't be the first one in line at the table, either. Slow down, enjoy yourself, and let people help themselves before you choose something to eat. Hopefully if you've had an AppeSizer before the party, you're not famished and can wait until the line dwindles.

Go easy on the alcohol. Socializing, for many of us, includes drinking alcohol. And that's fine ... in moderation. But remember those drinks are high in calories. [See Sidebar, Drinks with Your Diet in Mind, on page 76] On average, an alcoholic drink contains about 150 calories, but order a large frozen daiquiri and you're drinking 500 to 800 calories. Yikes!

Make your first drink non-alcoholic like sparkling water, diet soda, or even tomato juice. In other words, pace yourself. Set a limit beforehand—say, two or three drinks—and stick to it. You'll enjoy yourself more (and you won't miss the headache the next day).

Forget "banking" calories. Many people try to "save" calories throughout the day before a big dinner or evening celebration.

This almost always backfires, as you're so hungry by the time the event arrives you make up for the calories you missed and then some. Eat the way you normally would—starting with breakfast, of course—and spread your calories throughout the day. Then, have a small, healthy snack—an AppeSizer—before heading out, so you're not starving when you arrive. A piece of fruit and cheese or even a half-sandwich will take the edge off your appetite.

HOLIDAY HEAVEN—OR IS IT HELL?

You probably know how fattening the holidays are, and for good reason. Not only is more high-calorie food around, but we also face office parties, year-end bashes, and holiday get-togethers. Besides that, you're likely to be stressed out, sleep-deprived, and struggling to meet work and family obligations.

An oft-cited study found the average weight gain over the holidays is only a pound or so. However, diet-minded people may gain more. A more recent study compared the behavior of people of average-weight and that of "successful losers," people who lost a significant amount of weight and kept it off for years. Even though the weight-loss group was *four times* more likely to maintain their regular exercise routine during the holidays, they still had a 39 percent chance of gaining 2.2 pounds or more by New Year's Eve—compared to 17 percent of the other group. In trying to maintain their weight loss, they may have restricted calories too severely, which set them up for overeating and weight gain. Or they may be more prone to gain weight since they've struggled with it in the past. Another study found healthy college students gained a pound, on average, over Thanksgiving alone.

No, a pound isn't a lot. But if you never get it off (and most people don't), that yearly pound adds up to 10 pounds or more over a decade—in addition to the inevitable weight gain most of us experience as we grow older. That's why you've got to arm yourself with a slew of techniques to stay on track. Using the previous party strategies will help you survive the holidays. But in addition, I want to suggest six techniques to help you not just survive, but thrive, this time of year.

Safeguard your environment. You can't do anything about the plates of Christmas cookies at work or at your kids' school holiday celebration, but you can control your environment at home. How? First, if you're preparing food at home, *don't* buy your favorites. In other words, if you can't resist cheesecake, buy fruitcake instead … and if you inhale eggnog, keep it out of your refrigerator. Your favorite relative sent you a giant box of chocolate? Have a couple and then toss it, or at least put the box out of sight, where you won't be tempted to eat candy every time you cruise through the kitchen. Put healthy foods in eyesight so you're more likely to grab those first.

Have a plan. You already know that the more people you eat with, the more you tend to consume. Throw a little family drama into the mix and you may find yourself eating even more.

You probably can't escape your family this time of year, whether it's a cranky teenager or a demanding mother-in-law, but you can devise a plan. Let's say your older sister obsesses over what you eat—or what you don't. If you know she'll be upset when you refuse her homemade dessert ("But I made it just for *you!*"), tell her you'll have one *small* piece of chocolate cake if you really want it. However, if you don't want it, hold your ground and refuse politely or offer to take some home for later. Also, make sure you have something you *can* eat at family functions and other events. Having even one healthy choice gives you something to eat more of while taking a few small bites of the more fattening stuff.

Make time for exercise. Yes, you're busy. But maintaining your regular exercise routine will decrease stress and make you less likely to put on weight. When it comes to weight, remember it's calories *in* and calories *out*. The more calories you expend through exercise and daily activity, the more you can take in.

Besides, exercise is a great way to relieve stress—and most of us need stress relief during this time of year. Plus, research shows that regular exercise may help moderate your appetite—which means you'll eat less than if you skip workouts for a month. Just keep in mind that most people, especially women, tend to overestimate the number of calories they burn during exercise, or treat themselves with a high-calorie reward after their workout. Make exercise a regular part of your routine, not a reason to order an extra-large dessert that evening.

Here's one more suggestion: when you feel overwhelmed, don't settle for your usual routine. Step it up with an extra-challenging workout. Boosting your intensity not only burns a few extra calories, it helps you leave stressors (family members, to-do lists, endless socializing, you name it) behind ... at least for a bit.

Take the focus off food. While the holidays may seem to center around food, it doesn't have to be that way. After all, we don't just sit down and eat. We talk. We laugh. We bond. We argue. We eat some more. Hmmm ... add the fact that in most cultures and families food is associated with love, this time becomes especially challenging when it comes to adjusting the way you eat. But it can be done.

Think of all the things you can do with your family and friends besides eat—really. You can bond in other ways. Create and decorate ornaments together. Go ice-skating, biking, or walking as a group. Have a family game night or play cards. Rent a batch of favorite holiday movies and watch them as a group. Yes, you can (and will) eat. It just shouldn't be all you do, holiday-wise.

Forget perfection. Holidays aren't the time to insist on sticking to a rigid diet. Plan on having a few splurges and you won't feel guilty or angry at yourself afterwards. A big part of socializing is eating, and if you refuse to swallow anything "special" or obsess over weight, you may feel resentful and cranky—not quite how you want to spend the holidays.

So, forget perfection. Shoot for "pretty good." That goes for the rest of the celebrations as well. You don't have to bake six kinds of Christmas cookies from scratch or nail your biggest ever year-end bonus to make sure the holidays are wonderful for you and your family. Accept that your expectations may be a little high, and instead of the perfect holiday decorations or the most fabulous, once-in-a-lifetime gifts, aim for pretty good ones instead.

Get enough pillow time. With holiday shopping and socializing added to your already-busy schedule, you may be tempted to skimp on shut-eye this time of year. Don't. Tired people are irritable, distracted, and spacey—and often hungrier as well. One study found that men who only slept for four hours consumed, on average, 559 calories more the next day than men who slept a full eight hours. Another study with women found those who slept the least (less than five or six hours per night) were significantly more likely to gain weight over time than women who slept seven hours or more.

Researchers aren't exactly sure of the connection between sleep patterns and weight (more about that in Chapter 8), but getting insufficient REM, or rapid eye movement, sleep (the time when you dream) may affect your body's natural circadian rhythms that control metabolism, resulting in feeling hungrier than usual the next day. Another sleep bonus: maintaining your usual sleep patterns helps you cope with seasonal stressors. And besides joy, family, and peace to all mankind, let's face it—this time of year is all about stress, isn't it?

Navigating Travel, Holidays and
Special Occasions: How Others Do It

Need a pep talk or some more ideas for handling the holidays, travel, and other special occasions? Here's how some people manage:

66 When I travel, sometimes I feel like I'm away from home, so I can eat whatever I want. However, lately I've been traveling with protein bars and it satisfies that chocolate craving, also gives me protein, and isn't terrible on the calories. 99

Angie, 35, stay-at-home mom of 3

66 My biggest challenge eating-wise with the holidays is the massive amount of food available and the number of occasions to eat it. I work hard throughout the year to maintain my weight, so I like to think of the holidays as my time to indulge, but the best bet is to keep everything in moderation. It's okay to drink the eggnog, just not five glasses of it. If I know we're going to several parties in one day, then I try to spread out my intake at the different parties, or choose to eat a meal at one and then only have a drink or a snack at the other. Keeping your fitness routine, if you have one, is key during this time. Plus, it helps you keep your healthy habit throughout the year and into the new one, eliminating your need to make a resolution to get back to the gym. 99

Jill, 28, corporate communications writer

66 Traveling is difficult. I often eat only a banana or energy bar for breakfast. I'll go for a veggie sandwich at Subway or a black bean burrito at one of the Fresh Mex places. I don't eat junk food and I don't like fast food places, so this makes things a lot easier. If I'm dining more formally I'll try to have pasta/raviolis, a veggie sandwich, or a salad with balsamic vinaigrette. 99

Sam, 55, professional writer

"It depends on the month. If it's a month I'm trying to eat better, I'll get chicken instead of a burger and I try not to eat fries with every meal. If it's a month when I'm working out, I'll get chicken and a salad ... but I still feel hungry. You have to eat out every night on the road, so I make an effort to work out even when I'm busy. When I was on the road for five weeks straight, I was working out very hard every night. That gave me the motivation to eat well when I was out."

Mark, 28, producer and freelance camera/sound operator

"I am Cajun French. If anyone has been to Louisiana, they know about the food culture. I have recipes that have been in our family for generations. Of course, many of them are not low in calories. My plan for the holidays is to be disciplined about eating in moderation. I love to bake. I bake sweets during the holidays for events, but I try not to overindulge.

Where I do cut back is casseroles. Unfortunately, in our family, casseroles contain creamy sauces with a lot of calories and sodium. For some reason, people love to make green bean casserole loaded with creamy soup mix, instead of fresh steamed green beans. I cut out or cut back on those high calorie dishes. Another thing my husband and I do: instead of eating at someone else's house (where we don't have control of the menu items), we plan to arrive for coffee and dessert. With that plan, we can control what we're eating for dinner and not arrive too hungry."

Kayla, 36, registered nurse, mother of 4

You now have all the tools you need to eat right when your time is tight. In the next chapter you'll learn more strategies that make for a healthier, happier life—and save you time as well.

TUNE IN, TUNE OUT:

Finding Some Slow in Your Life on the Go

❝My freshman year of college, I gained not the "freshman 15," but the freshman 45. Not fun at all. I started running and working out (and cut back on what I was eating) to get the weight off, and it worked. In my 20s, I worked out to maintain my weight and look good. In my 30s, I worked out to manage stress. I started my own business and went through years of infertility. Now, in my 40s, I'm a business owner and mom, busier than ever before. But I've kept running and lifting weights because I love the way it makes me feel. I have more energy, more patience, and feel much happier when I'm exercising regularly—and my weight has been stable since my early 20s, which is a huge plus.❞

Kelly, 43, business owner and mother of 2

Many of the strategies I've shared in the preceding chapters are simple to remember and implement. Turning them into habits requires a bit of time and effort, but once those habits are in place, you're eating healthier, saving time, boosting your productivity, and losing weight without even trying. What could be better?

By adopting these strategies, you've saved time and hopefully even created more time, while improving your nutritional intake. But what are you *doing* with that extra time? How are you spending it? While it's important to make smart food choices on the go, it's also important to "find the slow in your go." In other words, consciously choosing to fully enjoy your time—and your life.

Four major aspects of your lifestyle influence your weight and overall health. You may not think about, or even be aware of, their dramatic impact on the way you feel and live. I call those four influences:

- The Stress Factor;
- The Sweat Factor;
- The Sleep Factor; and
- The Sunshine Factor.

GET THE STRESS OUT: WHY IT'S BAD FOR YOU AND HOW TO FIGHT IT

In Chapter 1 you learned stress is one of the biggest challenges to eating better. In our culture it's ever-present and inescapable. A recent poll found one-third of women and one-quarter of men are "highly stressed," and the majority of both men and women feel they're not doing enough to manage their stress. Stress can be a tricky thing, because it creates a host of physical and emotional symptoms (ranging from moodiness and anxiety to migraines and backaches) that you may attribute to poor health, rather than trying to do too many things at once.

Many of us (four in ten women and three in ten men) turn to food for comfort. But stress may have an even bigger impact on your weight than simply making ice cream more appealing. When you feel stressed, your body produces more stress hormones like adrenaline and cortisol. And studies show an increased level of cortisol makes you more likely to create and store belly fat—the fat that pads your internal organs, raising your risk of heart disease while enlarging your waistline.

Here's the headline version of the story: the more stressed you are, the more likely you are to gain weight over the long run. A study of middle-aged men found those who had the most trouble dealing with stress were more likely to gain weight over a five-year period than men who handled stress better. (Not surprisingly, men who exercised infrequently and consumed the most calories at dinner were also more likely to gain weight over that time period.)

Worse yet, if you're already overweight, you may have a higher risk of gaining weight as a result of stress. A recent study found those with the highest body weight at the outset who also had increasing levels of stress were more likely to gain weight over the next ten years. Men's stress levels tended to be related to work and money issues; women's stress levels were related to work, family issues, personal concerns, and money issues.

The good news is stress management doesn't mean shucking your responsibilities and running away to live on a desert island, though that may sound good to you. You only need a few minutes now and then to employ stress management techniques, which can be simpler and quicker than you might think. Just five minutes of daily relaxation—like taking time to slow down and focus on your breathing—can result in an energy boost that will save you time and prevent chronic ailments over the course of your life. So it's not a waste of time, but an investment of time, to make managing stress a priority.

There are loads of stress management techniques to choose from. Some people thrive on intense workouts, while others prefer mind-body exercise like yoga or Pilates. Listening to music may help you escape from your cares, while your best friend may prefer watching a sitcom. You won't know what works for you unless you try it. Here are ten proven ways to better handle the stress in your life—without stressing over having to do it:

- *Stay connected.* Supportive relationships with friends, family members, or both, can help you deal with day-to-day stressors.

Everyone needs at least one good friend (preferably someone who makes you laugh) you can rely on when life gets rough. The great thing about social media sites like Facebook is that they let you stay connected with friends both near and far, but there's no substitute for getting together with a friend for a drink, or with the guys for a pickup basketball game.

- *Eliminate emotional vampires.* This is the exception to staying connected. Some people just sap your strength, emotional energy, and joy. They're emotional vampires. Get rid of them when you can, or at least limit your exposure to them if you work with them (or you're related to them).

- *Meditate ... or not.* Meditation is an excellent way to deal with stress, but it's not for everyone. If you've tried this and it didn't work for you, don't give up. Try yoga, which enhances the mind-body connection, or a guided meditation CD that will walk you through a progressive relaxation sequence. Or sit quietly in a comfortable position and think of a word like "calm" or "peace" to help quiet your mental chatter.

- *Get creative.* Research shows creativity produces happy brain chemistry, and you needn't be an award-winning artist to lose yourself in an artistic pursuit. Embracing your creativity can be as simple as singing in the shower, taking photos, coloring with your child, or trying a new recipe.

- *Breathe easy.* Just focusing on your breathing can immediately reduce tension. As you inhale, concentrate on completely filling your lungs so your abdomen swells like a balloon. Then exhale completely, pulling your belly in toward your spine. Breathe this way for five minutes—even two—and you'll feel a difference.

- *Grin and bear it.* This may sound goofy, but it works. When you're feeling wrung out, smile and think positive thoughts. Simply forcing yourself to laugh for one minute will improve your mood. If that's too much of a stretch, think of someone you love and focus on that feeling.

- *Tune in*. Music offers an immediate escape. Choose any music you enjoy and find a comfortable spot where you can relax, close your eyes, and focus. A study of open heart surgery patients showed those who listened to soothing music after the procedure had significantly higher relaxation levels than those who didn't. If it works for them, it can work for you.
- *Write it down*. At the end of the day, take a few minutes to record what's bothering you. Research shows that keeping a journal and writing about your feelings and ways to cope with difficulties can have a positive effect on your mood and help reduce stress.
- *Get rubbed the right way*. Massage improves your circulation, reduces pain, and relieves tension—and it feels good, too. Schedule a massage at the end of an insanely busy week, or treat yourself after accomplishing something special.
- *Work it out*. When your stress levels skyrocket, breaking a sweat is one of the best ways to fight back. A gentle walk may not have as powerful an effect as more intense exercise, so shoot for a twenty-minute workout where you're breathing hard for more tension-reducing benefits.

These techniques are intended to give you ideas that may work for you, but feel free to come up with your stress-management methods as well. If curling up with a mug of tea and surrounding yourself with scented candles does the trick, so be it. If you'd rather surf YouTube for entertaining videos, that's fine too. The key is not *what* you do to relieve stress, but that you do it regularly—even when you don't feel stressed. That will make it easier for your body to handle day-to-day tensions without wreaking havoc on your waistline, mood, and health.

THE SWEAT FACTOR

Don't worry—you don't have to actually sweat buckets, but you do need to move, and move regularly. Besides how you eat, the way you move is the most important thing you can do to live better. That's why exercise gets its own Master Strategy—"sweat 30+."

Not only is exercise one of the most effective ways to help you manage stress, staying active also helps reduce your risk for nearly every medical condition you can think of. Plus it will boost your mood, alleviate depression, ease anxiety, and contribute to overall self-esteem and well-being.

This gives you plenty of reasons to work out, or at least find ways to add activity to your life. But an active lifestyle is also one of the most effective ways to keep extra weight off in the long run. One major study found those who exercised the most gained less weight than their more sedentary peers. Another recent study of nearly 5,000 men and women, found that over time, men and women gained, on average, 2.2 pounds a year. However, the more active ones weighed less than their couch potato peers. For example, women who walked for thirty minutes a day gained half as much weight over fifteen years as women who didn't walk for exercise.

Still, finding time to exercise can be a challenge. If you don't have an extra hour for the gym, don't give up. Instead, focus on the things you can do. Researchers find that performing even brief bursts of activity (say, a brisk ten-minute walk three times a day) is as good health-wise as a thirty-minute walk. And taking activity breaks throughout the day will stimulate your metabolism and give you a natural energy boost.

Here are 10 more ways to get more active, and enjoy it:

Walk away. Walking is the number one fitness activity for Americans. It's simple, easy, and all you need is a sturdy pair of comfortable shoes and appropriate clothing. Even a brief walk will improve your circulation, get more oxygen flowing to your brain, and clear your head. Walking may also temporarily decrease your appetite or help you beat a bad-for-you craving. Step outside for a quick stroll, or head for the stairs in your office for a couple of minutes.

Save your gas. If you drive to work, leave your car five blocks away from the office and walk the difference. If you have time, increase the distance for longer walking sessions. If you take the train or bus, get off at an earlier stop.

Take the long way. When you head to the bathroom or go for a cup of coffee, take the longest route possible, or add a few quick laps around the office before you return to your desk.

Use the stairs. Avoid the elevator whenever possible and opt for the stairs. If you work on the 30th floor, try getting off on the 25th floor instead. And if it's only a flight or two, the stairs are faster than waiting for the elevator anyway.

Think long-term. Exercise isn't fun for most people, at least not at first. But keep at it and you'll notice a difference in how you look and how you feel about yourself. One recent study found obese women who started an exercise and nutrition information program not only lost weight—they experienced significant improvements in mood, body image, and self-efficacy, or their belief in their own abilities.

Make it fun. Tennis, yoga, walking, golf--find your exercise of choice. This sounds obvious, but if you enjoy what you're doing, working out stops feeling like a chore and becomes something you'll look forward to—even if you've had trouble sticking to an exercise routine in the past.

Count your steps. Aim for 10,000 steps a day to reap the health benefits of being active. Strap on a pedometer to measure how active you are during the day and you'll see how close you come to that number. Strive to increase the number by 500 a day until you make the 10,000 per day goal.

Tune into tunes. Upbeat music can give you an immediate emotional boost, and research shows listening to music while you exercise makes your effort feel easier. Slipping on headphones (keep the volume down to protect your ears) is a great way to make your routine fly by. Use your Ipod or MP3 player to make motivating mixes that keep you going.

Change it up. How do you spend your typical day? A workout opposite your normal daily routine may be the most enjoyable for you. If your job entails running around for a demanding boss, you

How Do They Do It?

Besides eating right, getting and staying active will have the most dramatic impact on your body, energy level, mood, health, and self-esteem. But you know it takes time and effort to get your body off the couch. Read on to learn how real people—busy people like you—fit workouts into their lives:

> **"**When I need a boost of energy, I get up from my desk and take a lap around the office floor. Water, exercise, and healthy snacks have helped improve my overall health and focus at work. **"**
>
> *Cassandra, 38, transportation planner*

> **"**I look at my time at the gym as time for me. I've been trying to keep in my mind as I age that my body is a machine and needs adequate fuel to keep running in top-notch shape. As I age, working out becomes more important for stamina, energy, and just staying happy. It's all in your frame of mind, and living life to the fullest. You can't do that with a tired, sore, worn-out body. **"**
>
> *Sue, 50, stay-at-home mom of 3*

> **"**I typically run five days per week and lift weights at the gym twice a week. I run one or two marathons a year. This helps me stay in shape physically and mentally. It reduces my stress level and gives me more energy. **"**
>
> *Sam, 53, professional writer*

may want to try an activity where no one is telling you what to do—like vegging out on an elliptical trainer. But if you're self-employed and work alone, you may enjoy a group weight-lifting class or pickup basketball game where you get lots of social interaction and you don't have to figure out what to do.

66 It took me two years to knock off 20 extra pounds and I've kept it off for almost four years now. I created my own lifestyle change, and eating right and exercise kept me at this size. When I started, I walked thirty minutes; now I'm up to fifty minutes. On top of that, I use 5-pound weights while watching a cardio DVD or Fit TV. The combination varies depending on the week, but it's three to four times a week. Every so often I reward myself with a cheat day (eat anything I want) and maybe a treat like a new pair of shoes. 99

Colleen, 38, educator

66 For me, making time to work out is a mindset. I have a stressful job so I use exercise as a type of stress reliever. I know exercise is good for both the body and the mind. If I use that time to relieve stress, it makes me think clearer, which also allows me to concentrate more. This not only benefits me, but my team at work as well. At my job, if I'm not at my best, cases don't get closed and people can get hurt. That's exactly why I eat and exercise the way I do. Making sure people stay safe motivates me—I can't do that if I'm not taking care of myself. 99

Ryan, 36, police officer/Army

Target your heart. Using a heart rate monitor is a great way to add motivation to a program and get you out of a rut. This device straps around your chest to measure your heart rate and tell you how hard you're working. By using a monitor, you can ensure you're exercising intensely enough for health benefits, and keep yourself from overtraining as well. Plus you'll have concrete evidence you're getting fitter—as your heart gets stronger, your average heart rate will go down.

Try something new. Even if you're not usually a fitness class person, you now have more choices than ever before. You can sign up for a calorie-blasting class like spinning or kickboxing, or take a lower-key hatha yoga class to stretch and relax. If your schedule's too unpredictable for a regular class, invest in a few workout tapes to keep at home. Mastering new moves keeps your brain engaged, which keeps you from getting bored.

Find a buddy. Make a commitment to work out with another person and you'll be more likely to stick to your program. Find a like-minded co-worker or neighbor to exercise with, or join a local running or walking group.

Remember, you're in this for the long haul. I'd rather have you commit to something reasonable—say, making an effort to park further away from the store when you run errands, taking the stairs more often, and hitting the gym a couple of times a week—than launch an all-out seven-day-a-week exercise program you can't maintain for more than a few days. The key is to get—and stay—more active in a way that fits your lifestyle.

SLEEPLESS IN SEATTLE—AND SACRAMENTO, AND SPRINGFIELD

Do you awaken every morning wishing you had another precious hour of shut-eye? Do you often stay up late to finish work or household chores? Millions of us sacrifice sleep, not realizing we may also be sacrificing our health and well-being. Getting enough rest is more than a luxury. Simply put, sleep keeps you healthy—and helps you maintain a healthy weight as well.

A six-year study found those who slept the least (five to six hours per night) gained more weight over the next six years than those who slept seven to eight hours a night, or those who slept nine to ten hours. Recall the study I mentioned last chapter: even one night's poor sleep made people consume more than 500 extra calories the next day. That kind of extra intake can add up fast—a pound a week, in fact.

Experts still aren't sure why sleep is so essential to good health, but we know that during sleep our bodies repair and grow new tissue, produce less stress hormones like cortisol and adrenaline, and produce essential growth hormone. Sleep also helps regulate appetite and immune function.

Yet a national poll found only about 40 percent of Americans are getting a good night's sleep most nights—and that means 60 percent of us aren't sleeping well. While sleep needs vary, 30 percent of us are getting fewer than six hours of sleep each night, far short of what most people need for overall health and productivity.

We do know that when you're short on sleep, mental performance and mood suffer. A recent study found those who slept less than six hours the night before had higher depression, anxiety, and stress, and reported significantly poorer well-being than those who slept more than six hours. The poor sleepers also made more errors on simple cognitive tests and had a higher heart rate than the better sleepers. Another study found those who slept less than six hours did worse on a number of neuropsychological tests than those who slept more than six hours. And another study found poor sleep quality was linked to a significantly worse mood during the day. A bad mood? That's one thing. But taken too far, extreme sleep deprivation can cause cardiovascular complications and even death.

The Right Amount of Sleep

Don't look at sleep as something you have to do. Consider it an investment in the next day's mood, energy, and productivity. While according to the National Sleep Foundation, average adults need seven hours and twenty-four minutes a night, you may need as little as six hours a night, or even as much as nine hours per night, depending on factors like your diet, health, and activity level. The clue to whether you're getting enough is waking up refreshed every morning. If not, you're either not getting enough sleep—or not getting quality sleep.

Make sleep a priority; commit to getting more of it. To fall asleep more quickly and get better quality sleep, try these five strategies:

- *Be consistent.* Go to bed and get up at the same time every day, even on weekends. This will help you establish and maintain a healthy sleep habit.
- *Watch your diet.* Avoid caffeine, alcohol, and sugar six hours before you go to bed. All can make it harder to fall asleep and stay asleep.
- *Keep your bedroom separate.* Use your bed for sleep (and sex) alone. If you wake in the night and can't fall back to sleep, move to a different room to read or watch TV.
- *Exercise regularly.* The more active you are, the deeper sleep you get in general. But don't work up a sweat several hours before bedtime as that can make it harder to fall asleep.
- *Get comfortable.* Keep your room cool, dark, and quiet. Too-warm temperature, sound, and light can all interrupt your slumber.

Occasional insomnia is common, but if you have trouble falling asleep or staying asleep for more than two weeks or if you frequently awaken without feeling refreshed—and you're not skimping on sleep—seek medical advice from a sleep specialist.

THE SUNNY SIDE OF THE STREET

Finally, let's talk about attitude ... your own. How happy are you, overall? And do you know what's most likely to make you feel good in the long run? Factors like beauty, fame, and fortune are not the real keys to happiness. Experts say—and research proves—that even simple things can improve your personal "sunshine factor."

According to happiness researchers, two attributes are essential for day-to-day contentment: good mental health and positive social relationships. Good mental health means more than not feeling anxious or depressed; it also involves how you see the world (i.e., in a positive rather than negative light). True self-esteem— feeling good about yourself—means accepting who you are and not holding yourself to unrealistic standards.

I already talked about the importance of strong social relationships for stress management. Not surprisingly, they're the other most important aspect of happiness. Truly happy people have intimate relationships with people they care about—and who care about them in return. There's a health bonus as well. Research confirms that the more relationships a woman has, the healthier she's likely to be. (The effect isn't as pronounced for men.)

You may be surprised by another aspect to happiness. By following the Master Strategies and revamping your eating habits over time, you'll lose weight. And that's likely to have a positive impact on how you feel day to day, especially if you're a woman. A study with women found happiness was correlated with body esteem, and positive body image was a major contributor to overall happiness. What else can you do to be happier overall? Plenty. Give these ten strategies a try:

Watch a comedy you like. Laughing makes you feel good— even if you have to force it. One study found adults who forced themselves to laugh for just one minute felt significantly happier than those who didn't. Look for ways to get more laughter into your life and you'll feel happier overall.

Spend time with people you enjoy. Make time for your friends—especially those who make you laugh and "get" you. Having a lot of friends or an extended family may not be as important to your happiness as the quality of those relationships. In other words, a few close friends may be better for you than a dozen acquaintances. The key is how connected you feel—and how connected you want to be.

Spend money on someone else. A recent study found people who were randomly assigned to spend money on others experienced more happiness than those who were told to spend the money on themselves. If money is tight, random acts of kindness work just as well.

Set a goal—and go after it. Pursuing goals that are important to you give life meaning and improve overall happiness. The goal itself doesn't matter (say, writing a novel, learning how to sing opera, or traveling to China); what matters is its significance to you.

Make time for hobbies. If you have time for activities you enjoy, or you love your work (at least most days), you're likely to be happier than someone whose day is full of "must-dos" with little free time. Yet activities we do simply for pleasure tend to get dropped to the bottom of our to-do list. If you want to feel happier, make time for the things you love best, whether watching your favorite TV show, working in your yard, or playing with your dog.

Want what you have. Research shows the happiest people are those who have what they want—and want what they have. Focusing on what you have rather than what you don't have will make you more satisfied and happier overall than people who always compare themselves to others and come up short.

Work up a sweat. That's right, I'm talking about exercise again. Plenty of research attests to exercise's impact on short-term mood, but it lasts longer than that. One study of twins found those who exercised were more satisfied with their lives and happier, compared to non-exercisers.

Volunteer for a cause. Research shows that people who volunteer are happier than those who do not. Volunteering may increase empathetic emotions and help you appreciate what you have.

Have more sex. A recent review study found a clear association between sexual activity and satisfaction and emotional well-being, as well as overall quality of life for women. In other words, if you're happy with your sex life, you're likely to be happy with your overall life. Ask any guy, and he'll tell you the same thing.

Do what makes you happy. According to a recent survey, women listed rest and relaxation (66 percent), entertainment (61 percent), and a family meal (55 percent) as the top three activities that make them happy. Men listed entertainment (61 percent), rest and relaxation (60 percent), and digital entertainment (52 percent) as their top three. My point? Do what makes you happy, but don't expect your significant other to share exactly the same priorities. (Fortunately, both sexes listed "quality time with their partner" as their fourth favorite activity.)

These influences—stress, exercise, sleep, and attitude—impact your life every day, whether you're aware of it or not. Just as changing the way you eat will make a difference in your weight, mood, and health, making small changes in the way you live will do the same thing. In the end, you'll have more time to enjoy a slimmer, healthier, happier, more energetic *you*. And that's what eating right (and living right!) when time is tight is all about … and what I wish for you.

MEAL PLANS

for Typical (and Not-so-Typical) Days

In the previous chapters, you learned about the 10 Master Strategies and dozens of other ways to eat right when time is tight, including suggestions for all three meals and snacks. You've even got strategies for handling special occasions like business travel, vacations, and the holidays. But what about pulling it all together?

While I don't like diets that tell what to eat (and not eat) sometimes my clients want (or need) a more structured plan to follow. In the following pages you'll find meal plans for a variety of specific situations to make what you'll eat a no-brainer. Most meal plans include an optional dessert for when you're craving a little something extra. (Just remember, the idea isn't to follow the plan to the very letter, but to follow it in spirit and make it work for you.)

BLOWN-IT-AT-BRUNCH MEAL PLAN

Pancakes and sausage and eggs, oh my! It's one of those days where you've eaten way too much, and possibly even used up your entire fat and calorie allotment for the day ... and it's not even noon. You feel guilty, bloated, and out of control. What do you do now?

You may think you'll starve yourself for the rest of the day (which never goes well) or maybe you'll just give in to that voice in your head calling you a couch potato and hit the sofa for an afternoon nap. First, stop bashing yourself. The reality is that everybody overeats now and again. It's what you do afterwards that's important.

This meal plan will help you get back on track fast with low-calorie, hydrating foods to fill you up without weighing you down. Because you ate a large breakfast later in the morning, there will be no snacks today, but make sure you still "energize in 3-5" (Master Strategy 8) by eating lunch and dinner within five hours of each other. Another excellent strategy for days like today is to double up on your exercise. Not only will you burn more calories, you'll get an endorphin rush to help you feel energized and back in control.

Breakfast/Brunch

No idea; just waaaaay too much!

Late Lunch

Soup's On:
1 bowl (2 cups) low-sodium soup with beans and vegetables
1 seasonal fresh fruit
12 almonds

Snack Swap

Sweat 30+ and Hydrate:
Do an additional 30 minutes of exercise—even a half-hour stroll counts!
Additional 12 ounces of water with lemon, orange or cucumber slices

Dinner

Big Salad:
1 large bowl of mixed salad greens topped with
1 cup fresh veggies (e.g., tomatoes, cucumbers, carrots, celery, bell peppers)
3 ounces canned chunk-light tuna or other lean protein
1 ounce soft cheese (e.g., goat or feta cheese) or ½ ounce chopped nuts
2 tablespoons balsamic vinaigrette

CARPOOL-CRAZY DAY MEAL PLAN

When you've got kids to feed and errands to do, where can you find time to eat at all, let alone eat well? "Energize in 3-5" (Master Strategy 8) with your ER Survival Stash to fuel up and fight stress during a hectic weekday. Refined carbohydrates make your blood sugar levels peak and crash, soon leaving you hungry and irritable, but slow-digesting carbohydrates keep levels steady. Munching on a mix of protein (like hummus and nuts) and whole-grains, beans, and veggies throughout the day can clear your head, steady your hands, and allow you to focus on your to-do list.

Many of the same foods that keep your blood sugar stable and your stomach full also work as stress-busters. Walnuts are full of omega-3 fatty acids for healthy brain function and memory (if you can remember where you left the keys, you won't have to stress out looking for them!), and B-vitamins that are linked to good mental health. Avocados and bananas are high in potassium that helps naturally lower blood pressure. And the carbohydrates in whole-wheat muffins and pitas are related to higher tryptophan levels, which may help release serotonin, "the happiness hormone."

Breakfast

Nut-n-Honey Muffin:
1 whole-wheat English muffin
2 tablespoons all-natural nut butter
1 teaspoon of honey
1/2 banana, sliced on top

Snack (from ER Survival Stash)

Bar It:
1 whole-food bar [See Sidebar, Get the Most Energy from Your Energy Bar, page 107]

Lunch

Power Pita:
1/2 whole-wheat pita
1/3 avocado, sliced

3 slices (3 ounces) natural deli meat
Plus any fresh veggies you have handy that you can throw on!

Snack (from ER Survival Stash)

Trail Mix:
200-calorie trail mix snack pack (try Trader Joe's pre-portioned
  bags)

Dinner

Fast Family Feast:
1 rotisserie roast chicken (4-ounce servings each)
2 hot vegetable sides each; make one of them a green veggie
  and opt for steamed, baked or grilled options
1/2 cup applesauce each, with cinnamon on top

Dessert

Strawberries-n-Crème:
1 cup plain, low-fat Greek yogurt
1 teaspoon honey
1 teaspoon balsamic vinegar
1 cup fresh strawberries on stems
-   Mix yogurt with honey and vinegar. Serve as a dip with fresh
    strawberries on stems.

BEAT THAT COLD! MEAL PLAN

While there's no substitute for snoozing in pajamas, fluids from soup, frozen fruit bars, and tea help soothe your sore throat and flush out toxins. Bonus: foods rich in vitamin C and zinc may lessen the duration of your cold. If your appetite is low, focus on staying hydrated. If you can eat a little more, try a few small meals throughout the day to keep your body armed and your defenses strong.

No one knows why, but your grandmother's tried-and-true chicken soup remedy helps fight colds. Strengthen your immune system with fluids, electrolytes, protein, and vitamins to give you the strength to fight the nasty germs—and keep them from coming back.

Breakfast

Berry Smoothie:

1 cup low-fat, plain yogurt
1/2 cup fresh or frozen berries
1/2 cup 100 percent apple juice
1/2 cup crushed ice
- Blend until smooth.

Snack

Fruit & Cheese:

1 small citrus fruit
1 small piece of cheese (e.g., The Laughing Cow Mini Babybel)
8-ounce glass of water flavored with 100 percent juice or lemon
   or lime slices

Lunch

Tried-and-True Chicken Soup:

1 bowl (2 cups) low-sodium chicken rice soup
5 whole-grain crackers
1 mug of tea with honey and lemon

Snack

Nutty Squares:

1 full-sheet graham cracker (4 squares)
1 tablespoon all-natural nut butter
1 mug of tea with honey and lemon

Dinner

Avocado Scramble:

2 scrambled eggs with 1/2 avocado sliced on top
1 slice whole-wheat toast with 1 teaspoon butter and/or
   100 percent fruit spread
1 cup 100 percent fruit juice

Dessert

Fruit Up:

1/2 cup all-natural fruit sorbet or frozen fruit bar
   (e.g., Whole Fruit brand)
1 small handful almonds (10-12)
1 mug of tea with honey and lemon

SLEEPLESS NIGHT MEAL PLAN

Stress, insomnia, a new baby, a big night out—there are many reasons you may be getting less sleep than you need. Unfortunately, feeling tired the next day isn't the only consequence of getting too few ZZZZs. When you don't get enough sleep, your body tinkers with your hormone levels, altering your sense of hunger and satiety. Sleep deprivation causes levels of the hormone leptin (that tells your brain, "I'm full") to drop, and the hormone ghrelin (that tells your brain, "I'm hungry") to rise. That means you'll be hungrier than usual and have trouble knowing when you're full. If that weren't bad enough, you'll likely crave unhealthy, quick-digesting carbohydrate comfort foods like cheese pizza, doughnuts, and French fries.

While you can't tweak your hormone levels, you can adjust your diet. First, focus on healthy protein for breakfast when your carb cravings are the weakest. As the day progresses, turn to slow-digesting carbs. Pair those carbs with protein (Master Strategy 1) to satisfy your cravings, keep you fuller longer, and control your blood sugar levels. Instead of pasta or pizza for dinner, try substituting a hearty stew with potatoes or bean chili to sate the craving without overloading on empty calories.

Breakfast

Egg Sandwich:
1 scrambled or sliced hard-boiled egg
1 slice of cheese (organic if possible)
1 fistful of leafy greens (like arugula)
1 small whole-grain roll
- Toast roll if desired, and place egg, cheese, and greens to make the sandwich.

Snack

Hummus-Top Tomato:
1 large tomato, halved
¼ cup hummus or other bean-based dip
1 squirt of lemon
- Slice the tomato in half, top with hummus and finish with lemon juice.

Lunch

Asian Chicken Wrap:
1 large cabbage or lettuce leaf
1 cup shredded rotisserie chicken breast
1 fistful of fresh mung bean sprouts (or shredded cucumber or carrot)
2 teaspoons of peanut satay sauce
- Stuff chicken and sprouts in cabbage or lettuce leaf, drizzle with satay sauce and wrap.

Snack

Reboot:
Skip the snack and take a nap. If that's not possible, at least take ten minutes to close your eyes and mentally recharge. If you're still craving something sweet, have a frozen 100 percent fruit bar or 1 ounce (2 small squares) dark chocolate.

Dinner

Chili Out:
2 cups canned turkey or vegetarian chili (organic if possible)
1 cup frozen veggies
2 tablespoons natural, shredded extra sharp cheddar cheese
Fresh parsley or cilantro to taste (optional)
- Heat chili and mix with microwaved, frozen veggies. Top with shredded cheese and, if desired, fresh parsley or cilantro to taste.

Dessert

Hot Cocoa:
1 mug of hot chocolate with low-fat milk

PMS MEAL PLAN

Bloated? Frazzled? Wish you could stay in pajamas all day and eat pizza and ice cream? It must be that time of the month. Resist the chips; salt makes you retain water, which makes you feel bloated and puffy. Melons, cucumbers, and celery, are full of water, and act as a diuretic to flush salt out of your body. Potassium-rich avocados and bananas pack an extra punch. Drink lots of water today along with fiber-rich foods like dried plums and nuts to keep your GI tract moving and banish that bloat.

When choosing fruits and vegetables today, avoid cruciferous vegetables like broccoli, cauliflower, cabbage, and brussel sprouts, which can cause gas and discomfort. And to combat PMS mood-swings, munch on whole-grain carbohydrates like waffles or whole-wheat bread or tortillas that contain tryptophan, a building block of serotonin. Serotonin is a neurotransmitter best known for its mood-lifting properties.

Breakfast

Waffle Wise:
2 low-fat, whole-grain frozen waffles
   (about 80-100 calories each)
1/2 cup fresh or thawed, unsweetened frozen berries
1 tablespoon nuts (3-5)
1 tablespoon maple syrup
- Toast waffles and top with berries and syrup.

Snack

Red Ants on a Log:
Celery sticks topped with
1 tablespoon all-natural nut butter and
8-10 dried tart cherries

Lunch

Spicy Avocado Delight:
1/2 soft avocado
1 cup plain, nonfat Greek yogurt
Spicy seasoning to taste
1 slice dark brown bread
2 slices (2 ounces) natural, low-sodium turkey
10 thin slices of cucumber
- Mash avocado with yogurt and seasoning. Spread on bread and top with turkey and cucumber slices. Eat open-faced.

Snack

Melon-cotta:
1 slice melon
1/4 cup reduced-fat ricotta cheese
Pinch of cinnamon or cardamom
1 full-sheet graham cracker (4 squares)
- Slice melon, top with ricotta cheese and a pinch of cinn-amon or cardamom. Enjoy with 1 full-sheet graham cracker.

Dinner

Tuna Tortilla:

1 can (4 ounces drained) water-packed light tuna
2 tablespoons balsamic vinaigrette
1 whole-grain tortilla
2 cups sliced vegetables (e.g., cucumbers and carrots)
- Mix drained tuna with dressing, fold into tortilla along with sliced vegetables.

Dessert

Pistachios & Chocolate:

30 pistachios
1 tablespoon dark chocolate chips

BIG PRESENTATION DAY MEAL PLAN

Stave off presentation day jitters with a breakfast loaded with high-fiber whole-grains, low-fat dairy, and fruits. You might be tempted to skip breakfast when you're anxious, but an empty stomach will only cause blood sugar levels to plummet, leaving you tired and light-headed. Plus studies show (remember Chapter 3) that breakfast may improve short-term memory and attention.

For an added mental boost, include omega-3 rich foods (e.g., salmon, walnuts, seaweed, and olive oil) for brain function, anti-oxidant-rich berries (e.g., cranberries, blackberries, and blue-berries); caffeine to make you more alert (limit to 1 or 2 cups a day; too much can make you jittery and uncomfortable); and a bit of dark chocolate (yes chocolate!), which has antioxidants and natural stimulants like caffeine to enhance focus and concentration.

In addition to your diet, ensure you ace your presentation by remembering to get a good night's sleep. Staying hydrated, getting a quick morning workout in (to help sharpen your thinking), and taking time to meditate or simply taking a few deep breaths beforehand (to clear your head and relax) will also help you perform optimally on that all-important day.

Breakfast ....

Cereal & Fruit:
1-2 cups high-fiber cereal [See Sidebar, The Skinny
  on Breakfast Cereals, page 42]
1 cup nonfat milk or calcium-fortified soy milk
1 seasonal fresh fruit
1 mug coffee or tea
Added boost: morning exercise and/or meditation or
  deep breathing

Snack ....

Yogurt & Berries:
1 cup nonfat, plain yogurt
1/2 cup berries
Drizzle of honey (1 teaspoon)

Lunch (rushed at work, remember to eat!) ....

Burrito Boost:
1 organic frozen burrito heated in microwave
  (e.g., Amy's brand) with
Lots of fresh salsa
1/2 cup low-fat cottage cheese on the side

Snack ....

Reese's Right:
1/2 ounce dark chocolate (2 small squares)
1 small handful walnuts (1/2 ounce or 7 halves)

Dinner ....

Chicken Ease:
3/4 cup skinless, rotisserie chicken
1 cup cooked seasonal vegetables
1/2 cup organic microwave whole-grain rice
  (e.g., Seeds of Change microwavable rice and grains)

Dessert (celebrate!) ....

Fro-Yo Canapes:
2 whole-grain graham crackers
1/2 tablespoon all-natural nut butter
1/4 cup low-fat vanilla frozen yogurt
  -   Spread nut butter on graham crackers and
      top with frozen yogurt.

BOX LUNCH DAY MEAL PLAN

We all have days where we can't control what we have for lunch and simply have to eat what everyone else is having. A filling fiber- and protein-rich breakfast will keep your blood sugar levels steady until mid-morning snack time. Before lunch, enjoy a desk-time AppeSizer, a low-cal soup that will downsize your appetite for lunch. When you're confronted with brown boxes full of mayonnaise-laced sandwiches, try removing half the bread for an open-faced lunch, make a beeline for the fruit bowl, and choose either chips *or* a cookie for dessert. Let your big breakfast and filling soup carry you through this dieting disaster area until dinnertime.

Breakfast

Egg-lish Muffin Crostini:
1/2 toasted whole-grain English muffin
1 poached egg
1 slice lean ham
1 thin slice (1/2 ounce) Swiss cheese
 - Serve egg, ham, and cheese open-face on English muffin

Snack

AppeSizer:
1 cup low-sodium, broth-based soup
5 whole-grain crackers, crumbled

Lunch

Box Lunch:
1 non-mayonnaise based sandwich (if possible) OR
  1 open-faced mayonnaise-based sandwich
1 piece of fruit
Chips or cookie (optional)

Snack (from ER Survival Stash)

Trail Mix:
1 small handful dried fruit (1/2 ounce)
1 small handful walnuts (1/2 ounce or 7 halves)

Dinner

Big Salad:
1 large bowl of mixed salad greens topped with

1 cup fresh veggies (e.g., tomatoes, cucumbers, carrots,
  celery, bell peppers)
1/2 cup canned, rinsed beans (e.g., kidney or chickpeas)
1 ounce soft cheese (e.g., goat or feta cheese)
2 teaspoons dried cranberries
2 tablespoons balsamic vinaigrette

STARVING AT SIX MEAL PLAN

You practically lunge toward the refrigerator, ravenous after a
hectic day that left little time to eat. What can you do to curb your
urge to rip open a bag of snack food to sate that stomach-growling,
hand-shaking, light-headed feeling? Hunger, meet microwave.
Microwave, meet hunger. After you eat an AppeSizer, hit the
freezer and throw a bag of frozen stir-fry vegetables and brown rice
in the microwave. Heat up some pre-cooked chicken or shrimp.
Just a few minutes after you walk in the door, you'll be sitting down
to a piping hot, fiber-filled, protein-packed dinner.

All Day
Not enough; famished!

Snack
AppeSizer:
1 apple
1 small piece of cheese (e.g., The Laughing Cow Mini Babybel)

Dinner
Stir-fry Rescue:
2 cups frozen stir fry vegetables
1 small handful (2 tablespoons) chopped cashews (or any nuts)
3/4 cup microwave brown rice
4-5 ounces pre-cooked shrimp (or any leftover grilled lean
  meat, fish, or poultry)
1 tablespoon low-sodium soy sauce or stir-fry sauce
- Heat brown rice and vegetables separately in microwave.
   Mix with heated shrimp (or other lean meat) and chopped
   nuts. Top with low-sodium soy sauce.

Dessert
Greek Yogurt & Jam:
1/2 cup plain, low-fat Greek yogurt mixed with
1 tablespoon 100 percent fruit spread/jam of choice

FAMILY ROAD TRIP MEAL PLAN

While family road trips can be unpredictable ("I thought you said we had a spare tire!"), your meals don't have to be. Navigate the open road with a compass pointed toward healthy meals and snacks from fast food restaurants and gas station pit stops. At lunch and dinner time, look for lean meats and entrees labeled as "grilled," "char-grilled," "broiled," "steamed," or "roasted." For snack time, just reach into your ER Survival Stash for hunger-busting whole-food bars, dried fruit, nuts, and whole-grain crackers.

Breakfast (at home)
Oatmeal Yum:
1 cup oatmeal topped with each:
2 tablespoons chopped nuts
2 tablespoons dried fruit
Pinch of cinnamon
Drizzle of honey (1 teaspoon)

Snack (from your ER Survival Stash)
Fruit Up:
1 serving of apple slices or 1 ounce dried fruit (1/4 cup)
1 small piece of cheese (e.g., The Laughing Cow Light Wedge)

Lunch (fast food stop)
Fast Wrap:
1 grilled chicken wrap or soft taco

Snack (gas station stop)
Seeds Please:
1 handful (1 ounce) of roasted sunflower seeds

Dinner (casual restaurant)
Veg Out:
1 cup of broth-based soup with beans and vegetables
Fish or chicken with a double side of vegetables

Dessert (from your ER Survival Stash)
Nuts & Chocolate:
1 small handful nuts (10-12)
1/2 ounce dark chocolate (1 small square)

FAMILY FETE MEAL PLAN

You're surrounded ... by friends, family, and food. Lots of food. That wide variety of food (plus that drink in your hand) doesn't just make your mouth water—it makes it hard to resist falling off the wellness wagon. Since parties should be about having a great time with loved ones, not stressing over calories, map out a healthy pre-party meal plan and then enjoy the evening!

The most important thing to do when you wake up the morning of a big party is to eat. That may sound counterintuitive, but remember to "munch every morn" (Master Strategy 3) because skipping meals during the day may lead to binge eating at night. Don't save your calories for phyllo-wrapped spinach puffs; instead, eat healthy food to stabilize your blood sugar levels, and fill up with water so you'll be full of willpower by party time. If you have a small snack like a handful of nuts and dried fruit or a salad before the party, you may be less tempted by the hors d'oeuvres. Remember to opt for low-salt food during the day to reduce bloating so you look and feel your best at the party.

Breakfast

Egg-lish Muffin & Greens:
1 whole-wheat English muffin
1 cooked egg
1 slice cooked Canadian bacon
Watercress or baby spinach (or any leafy greens)
A squirt of lemon
- Toast English muffin and stuff with egg, Canadian bacon, and greens. Top with a squirt of lemon.

Snack

Hummus-cuc Sandwiches:
20 slices English cucumber
2 tablespoons hummus
- Cut cucumber slices. Spread hummus on 10 slices and top with remaining slices.

Lunch

Better Burger:

1 medium veggie or turkey burger (about 5 ounces)

1 whole-wheat bun

Mixed veggies for burger and side salad
(e.g., salad greens, tomato, onion, and cucumber)

2 teaspoons Dijon mustard

1-2 tablespoons balsamic vinaigrette

- Top your burger with veggies and Dijon mustard. Enjoy with a side salad and splash of balsamic vinaigrette.

Snack (right before party)

AppeSizer:

1 cup broth-based soup

1 apple

HIGH-IN-THE-SKY MEAL PLAN

Waking up early, wandering around the airport, and sitting on a plane for hours can leave you dehydrated and sluggish at your business meeting. Avoid the high-fat, tempting food that follows you from the terminal to your destination by bringing your own nonperishable snacks, and seeking out healthful airport options. If you don't have time to pack snacks at home, there are options at airport shops like sunflower seeds, whole-food bars, and soy chips ... some even have fresh fruit. When you have some time, find the drugstore near your hotel and stock up on healthy snacks for your room. Remember to drink lots of water—pressurized airplane cabins are dehydrating. Losing water and not replacing it can lead to difficulty concentrating, sluggishness, and even snack attacks as you confuse thirst and hunger signals.

Breakfast (at airport)

Egg-cellent Start:

Small egg and veggie omelet or small breakfast burrito

Side of fresh fruit (instead of hash browns or potatoes)

1 cup of coffee or tea with nonfat milk

Snack (at airport)

Get Crackin':

1 ounce in-shell pistachios (49 nuts)

Lunch (pick up at the airport for the flight)

Super Sandwich:
1 small turkey or vegetarian sandwich on whole-wheat bread
   with veggies (e.g., lettuce, tomato, and cucumbers)
1 mustard packet
1 small salad with vinaigrette dressing (light if possible)

Snack (a store near your hotel)

Bar It:
1 whole-food bar [See Sidebar, Get the Most Energy from Your
   Energy Bar, on page 107]

Dinner (casual restaurant near the hotel)

Grilled Salmon Salad:
1 cup of broth-based soup
Big salad topped with grilled salmon and 1-2 tablespoons balsamic vinaigrette

BUSINESS TRIP/HOTEL STAY MEAL PLAN

You've safeguarded your environment (Master Strategy 2) by "fat-proofing" your home, office, and car. You've cleaned out your kitchen and always have portion-controlled snacks on hand, and you feel completely comfortable and in charge of your healthy lifestyle. But no matter how organized and dedicated you are, business travel presents new challenges that are out of your control. From complimentary breakfast buffets to multi-course business dinners, you're presented with new foods – maybe some of your biggest temptations. The Master Strategies and a sample meal plan will help you navigate your business trip so you can focus on your work, not your weight.

Remember to wake up in time for breakfast and eat something that contains protein and fiber. Most buffets have hot oatmeal and at least one high-fiber cereal, so skip the muffins and bacon for the tried-and-true whole-grains. Take advantage of the portable offerings at breakfast and grab a piece of hand fruit like an apple or pear for your ER Survival Stash.

Safeguard your hotel room and rental car by stocking up on

snacks at a local drugstore or hotel shop where you'll likely find nuts, seeds, whole-food bars, all-natural peanut butter, and whole-grain crackers. If your room has a miniature fridge, take advantage of it! Consider stowing some cheese, hummus, and low-fat yogurt in there for greater snack variety.

At a multi-course dinner, remember to order a broth-based soup or salad AppeSizer—a starter that is low in calories and takes time to eat. That will give your stomach a chance to tell your brain that you're getting full. For dessert, stick with fresh fruit or share a decadent dessert with the table. Savor three small bites of that chocolate cake and then leave it for the others.

Breakfast (hotel breakfast bar)
Oatmeal & Fruit:
1 cup oatmeal with 2 tablespoons granola or nuts
1 small banana
- Grab an extra piece of fruit and low-fat yogurt for later

Snack (saved from breakfast bar)
Fruit & Yogurt:
1 piece of fruit
1 cup low-fat yogurt

Lunch (restaurant)
Sushi Love:
1 sushi roll (wrapped in brown rice if possible; stay away from menu items that say "spicy," "crunchy," or have sauce)
1/2 cup steamed edamame
1 cup miso soup

Snack (from ER Survival Stash)
Bar It:
1 whole-food bar [See Sidebar, Get the Most Energy from Your Energy Bar, on page 107]

Dinner (restaurant)
Chinese Delight:
1/2 cup stir-fried or steamed protein
   (e.g., shrimp, chicken, beef)
1 cup stir-fried or steamed mixed vegetables

1/2 cup steamed rice (brown if possible)
Splash of low-sodium soy sauce
- Stay away from fried menu items labeled "crispy" and those
  with a special sauce

BEACH DAY MEAL PLAN

Slipping into a bikini (or maybe a tankini) later today? Whether
you're hitting the beach or a pool party, look your best by munching
on water-filled fruits and vegetables and low-salt snacks. Stash a
bunch of thirst-quenching frozen grapes in your cooler and you'll
be surprised how creamy they taste by snack time (and how much
easier it is to turn down an ice-cream cone). As the sun starts to set
and you head back for dinner, crack open some naturally low-cal,
low-sodium shrimp with a refreshing citrus salad. With this filling,
no-bloat plan, you'll feel energized and look great from the sand to
the sack!

Breakfast

Morning Slim-Down:
1/2 grapefruit
1 hardboiled or scrambled egg
1 slice of whole-wheat toast with 1 teaspoon butter and/or
    100 percent fruit jam

Snack

Sassy Celery Sticks:
1 cup celery sticks topped with
2 tablespoons Neufchatel (light cream) cheese and
1 tablespoon chopped nuts

Lunch (pre-packed for beach)

Mini Italian Sub:
1 whole-grain roll topped with
1 ounce (2 slices) low-sodium prosciutto or lean ham
1 ounce part-skim mozzarella
1 teaspoon 100 percent apricot spread
1 large handful fresh baby greens (like baby arugula)
Enjoy with seasonal fresh fruit or 1/4 cup dried veggies

Snack (pre-packed for beach)

Frozen Grapes & Cheese:
1 cup frozen grapes
1 small piece of cheese (e.g., The Laughing Cow Mini Babybel)

Dinner

Grilled Shrimp Salad:
1 large bowl of greens topped with
4 ounces grilled shrimp
1/2 cup avocado chunks
1/4 cup soft cheese (e.g., goat or feta)
1 cup chopped vegetables of your choice
2 tablespoons balsamic vinaigrette

Dessert

Frozen Banana Treat:
1 frozen peeled banana topped with
1 tablespoon all-natural nut butter

GET IN TOUCH—AND STAY IN TOUCH

Has this book helped you eat better, lose weight, have more energy, and get more done—or do you have a great suggestion or technique that's worked for you that you'd like to share? I'd love to hear from you—send me an email at patricia@patriciabannan.com.

And if you'd like to know what I'm working on, follow me on twitter: @nutritiongogo or visit www.patriciabannan.com.

APPENDIX

Looking for more information about eating right, and living better, when time is tight? Check out the following resources:

NUTRITION/FOOD

- www.nutrition.gov - This USDA-sponsored site includes nutrition info as well as advice on weight management, shopping and cooking tips, and related links.

- www.nal.usda.gov/fnic/foodcomp/search - The USDA's Nutrition Data Laboratory lets you look up the nutrient profile of any food and serving size.

- www.hsph.harvard.edu/nutritionsource - Maintained by the Harvard School for Public Health, the Nutrition Source contains nutrition info, recent research, and recipes.

- www.organic.org - Provides information about organic foods as well as reviews of foods and other organic products.

- www.eatright.org - The American Dietetic Association's site provides nutrition and food information.

- www.edf.org - The Environmental Defense Fund's website includes a printable Seafood Pocket Guide and a Sushi Pocket Guide you can carry with you.
- www.bonnietaubdix.com - Bonnie Taub-Dix, MA, RD, CDN, is the author of *Read It Before You Eat It.* Her book provides information on reading and understanding food labels.
- www.biggreencookbook.com - Want to learn how to cook and eat eco-friendly? Check out the *Big Green Cookbook*, by Jackie Newgent, RD.

FITNESS/HEALTH

- www.healthetips.com - A premier provider of lifestyle information, Health-E-tips helps organizations and schools improve the wellness of their employees and students.
- www.healthierus.gov - This site provides information to help you create healthier habits and get more activity into your daily life.
- www.healthfinder.gov/prevention - A quick guide to healthy living from the US Department of Health and Human Services.
- www.eventsoftheheart.org - The nonprofit organization, Events of the Heart, uses the creative arts to help women unite for better heart health.
- www.familydoctor.org - This comprehensive site, operated by the American Academy of Family Physicians, lets you research health conditions and topics that affect people of all ages; you can even search by symptom.
- www.squeezeitin.com - This fun site gives you tips and products to help you stay fit no matter how busy you are.
- www.webmd.com - One of the best-known health websites, this is another excellent site to learn more about different health conditions and the latest in health news and research.

ABOUT THE AUTHOR

Patricia Bannan, M.S., R.D., a Los Angeles-based registered dietitian, specializes in nutrition and health communications. She develops news segments for television stations, writes articles for magazines, and serves as a consultant and spokesperson to PR agencies and industry groups nationwide.

Patricia has appeared as a guest expert on more than thirty news shows, including ABC, CBS, Fox, and NBC's *Today* show. She has written articles for such leading magazines as *Self* and *Shape* and has been interviewed by numerous print media, including *The New York Times*, *Newsday*, *People*, *Redbook*, and *Ladies Home Journal*. In the broadcast news arena, she worked as a freelance producer and correspondent for CNN's New York Bureau, where she developed daily news stories and assisted on "Your Health," CNN's weekend health show.

Passionate about helping children and adults implement easy steps to improve their lives, Patricia's creative and doable health messages reach six million people each day through the in-school and corporate wellness programs of Health-E-tips, Inc. As a public relations and food industry consultant, Patricia helps develop strategic platforms and oversees tactical execution for health professional, consumer, and media outreach programs.

She graduated cum laude from the University of Delaware with a Bachelor of Science in nutrition and dietetics and completed her dietetic training at the National Institutes of Health in Bethesda, Maryland. Patricia received a Masters of Science in nutrition communication from the Friedman School of Nutrition Science and Policy at Tufts University in Boston, Massachusetts.

Prior to Los Angeles, Patricia lived in New York City for several years. She is a native of Silver Spring, Maryland, located just ten miles outside our nation's capital.

BIBLIOGRAPHY

Chapter 1

Interview with Alice C. Domar, Ph.D., December 15, 2009.
Nutrition and You: Trends 2008, American Dietetic Association press release; www.eatright.org

Larger portion sizes lead to a sustained increase in energy intake over 2 days. Rolls BJ, Roe LS, Meengs JS. Journal of the American Dietetic Association. April 2006;106(4):543-9.

Caloric consumption stats from USDA, www.usda.gov

Expanding portion sizes in the US marketplace: implications for nutrition counseling. Young LR, Nestle M. Journal of the American Dietetic Association. February 2003;103(2):231-4.

Sleep curtailment is accompanied by increased intake of calories from snacks. Nedeltcheva AV, Kilkus JM, Imperial J, Kasza K, Schoeller DA, Penev PD. American Journal of Clinical Nutrition. January 2009; 89(1):126-33.

Acute partial sleep deprivation increases food intake in healthy men. Brondel L, Romer MA, Nougues PM, Touyarou P, Davenne D. American Journal of Clinical Nutrition. June 2010; 91(6):1550-9.

Short sleep deprivation and weight gain: a systematic review. Patel SR, Hu FB. Obesity (Silver Spring). March 2008; 16(3):643-53.

Association between reduced sleep and weight gain in women. Patel
SR, Malhotra A, White DP, Gottlieb DJ, Hu FB. American
Journal of Epidemiology. November 15, 2006; 164(10):947-54.

Environmental factors that increase the food intake and consumption volume
of unknowing consumers. Wansink B. Annual Review of Nutrition. 2004;
24:455-79.

Effect of ambience on food intake and food choice. Stroebele N, De Castro
JM. Nutrition. September 2004; 20(9): 821-38.

2008 Stress in America poll, American Psychology Association, www.
apa.org

Relationship between stress, eating behavior, and obesity. Torres SJ,
Nowson CA. Nutrition. November-December 2007;23(11-12):887-
94.

Statistics from the National Sleep Foundation, www.sleepfoundation.
org

Results from "What do Women Want?" survey, www.marketingcharts.
com/direct/women-more-concerned-about-diet-and-weight-than-
serious-diseases-4679/

Statistics from the Centers for Disease Control, http://www.cdc.gov/
obesity/data/

Prevalence and trends in obesity among US adults, 1999-2008. Flegal,
KM, Carroll MD, Ogden CL, Curtin LR. Journal of the American
Medical Association. 2010; 303(3):235-241.

Survey by Self magazine and University of North Carolina at Chapel
Hill; press release dated April 22, 2008; http://www.unchealthcare.
org/site/newsroom/news/2008/Apr/selfsurvey/

Chapter 2

Dietary Guidelines for Americans, 2005; http://www.health.gov/
dietaryguidelines/dga2005/document/default.htm

Dietary fiber and weight regulation. Howard NC, Saltzman E, Roberts
SB. Nutrition Review. May 2001: 59(5): 129-139.

Statistics from the National Weight Control Registry, www.nwcr.ws
Research/default.htm

Selective effects of acute exercise and breakfast interventions on mood
and motivation to eat. Lluch A, Hubert P, King NA, Blundell JE.
Physiology & Behavior. 2000; 68: 515-520.

Breakfast cereal and caffeinated coffee: effect on working memory, attention, mood and cardiovascular function. Smith AP, Clark R, Gallagher J. Physiology & Behavior. 1999; 67(1):9-17.

Vegetables, fruits and phytoestrogens in the prevention of diseases. Heber D. Journal of Postgraduate Medicine. April-June 2004; 50(2):145-9.

Physical exercise and health: a review. Adamu B, Sani MU, Abdu A. Nigerian Journal of Medicine. July-September 2006;15(3):190-6.

Testing causality in the association between regular exercise and symptoms of anxiety and depression. De Moor MH, Boomsma DI, Stubbe JH, Willemsen G, de Geus EJ. Archives of General Psychiatry. August 2008; 65(8):897-905.

Exercise barriers, self-efficacy, and stages of change. Simonavice EM, Wiggins MS. Perceptual Motor Skills. December 2008; 107(3):946-50.

Chapter 3

Fasting biases brain reward systems toward high-calorie foods. Goldstone AP, de Hernandez CG, Beaver JD, Muhammed K, Croese C, Bell G, Durighel G, Hughes E, Waldman AD, Frost G, Bell JD. European Journal of Neuroscience. October 2009: 30(8): 1625-35.

Associations between obesity, breakfast-time food habits and intake of energy and nutrients in a group of elderly Madrid residents. Ortega RM, Redondo MR, Lopez-Sobaler AM, Quintas ME, Zamora MJ, Andres P, Encinas-Sotillos A. Journal of the American College of Nutrition. 1996: 15(1): 65-72.

Selective effects of acute exercise and breakfast interventions on mood and motivation to eat. Lluch A, Hubert P, King NA, Blundell JE. Physiology & Behavior. 2000: 68: 515-520.

Breakfast cereal and caffeinated coffee: effect on working memory, attention, mood and cardiovascular function. Smith AP, Clark R, Gallagher J. Physiology & Behavior. 1999: 67(1):9-17.

Breakfast eating habit and its influence on attention-concentration, immediate memory and school achievement. Gajre NS, Fernandez S, Balakrishna N, Vazir S. Indian Pediatrics. October 2008; 45(10): 824-828.

Influence of having breakfast on cognitive performance and mood in 13- to 20-year-old high school students; results of a crossover trial. Weidenhorn-Muller K, Hille K, Klenk J, Weiland U. Pediatrics. August 2008: 122(2): 279-84.

Relationships between dietary habits and the prevalence of fatigue in medical students. Tanaka M, Mizuno K, Fukuda S, Shigihara Y, Watanabe Y. Nutrition. October 2008; 24(10): 985-9.

Elevating blood glucose level increases the retention of information from a public safety video. Morris N. Biology and psychology. May 2008: 78(2):188-90.

Stress, breakfast cereal consumption and objective signs of upper respiratory tract illnesses. Smith, AP. Nutritional neuroscience. 2002:5(2):145-148.

Breakfast, blood sugar, and cognition. Benton D, Parker PY. American Journal of Clinical Nutrition. April 1998;67(4):772S-778S.

Association of breakfast energy density with diet quality and body mass index in American adults: national Health and Nutrition Examination Surveys, 1999-2004. Kant AK, Andon MB, Angelopoulos TJ, Rippe JM. American Journal of Clinical Nutrition. November 2008; 88(5):1396-404.

Breakfast skipping and its relation to BMI and health-compromising behaviours among Greek adolescents. Kapantais E, Chala E, Kaklamanou D, Lanaras L, Kaklamanou M, Tzotzas T. Public Health Nutrition. June 2010; 8:1-8.

Statistics from the National Weight Control Registry, www.nwcr.ws/Research/default.htm

Comparison of prebiotic effects of arabinoxylan oligosaccharides and inulin in a simulator of the human intestinal microbial ecosystem. Grootaert C, Van den Abbeele P, Marzorati M, Broekaert WF, Courtin CM, Delcour JA, Verstraete W, Van de Wiele T. FEMS Microbiology Ecology. August 2009;69(2):231-42. www.mypyramid.gov

Caffeine (1, 3, 7-trimethylxanthine) in foods: a comprehensive review on consumption, functionality, safety, and regulatory matters. Heckman MA, Weil J, Gonzalez de Mejia E. Journal of Food Science. April 2010:75(3):R77-87.

Tea and health: the underlying mechanisms. Weisburger JH. Proceedings of the Society of Experimental and Biological Medicine. 1999;220:271-5.

Caffeine content from Center for Science in the Public Interest, http://www.cspinet.org/new/cafchart.htm

Survey conducted in 2006 of people's typical breakfasts; www.npd.com/press/releases/press_061212.html

Chapter 4

Stats on diet industry, http://www.businessweek.com/debateroom/archives/2008/01/the_diet_indust.html

Top 10 fast-food restaurants, the QSR 50, www.qsrmagazine.com/reports/qsr50/2007/charts/qsr50-1.phtml

Nutrition and You: Trends 2008, American Dietetic Association press release; www.eatright.org

The NPD Group's Twenty-Fourth annual Report on Eating Patterns in America, www.npd.com/EPA

Expanding portion sizes in the US marketplace: implications for nutrition counseling. Young LR, Nestle M. Journal of the American Dietetic Association. February 2003;103(2):231-4.

Soup preloads in a variety of forms reduce meal energy intake. Flood JE, Rolls BJ. Appetite. November 2007; 49(3):626-34.

Dietary Guidelines for Americans, 2005; http://www.health.gov/dietaryguidelines/dga2005/document/default.htm

Definition of "natural" and "organic," www.usda.gov

Antioxidant effectiveness of organically and non-organically grown red oranges in cell culture systems. Tarozzi A, Hrelia S, Angeloni C, Morroni F, Biagi P, Guardigli M, Cantelli-Forti G, Hrelia P. European Journal of Nutrition. March 2006; 5(3):152-8.

Phenolic content and antioxidant activities of white and purple juices manufactured with organically- or conventionally-produced grapes. Dani C, Oliboni LS, Vanderlinde R, Bonatto D, Salvador M, Henriques JA. Food Chemistry and Toxicology. December 2007; 45(12):2574-80.

Statistics on purchasing organic food, http://www.ota.com/organic/mt/consumer.html

Background on organic foods, "Organic Foods-Overview," www.webmd.com/diet/tc/organic-foods-overview?print=true

Chapter 5

Situational effects on meal intake: a comparison of eating alone and eating with others. Hetherington MA, Anderson AS, Norton GN, Newson L. Physiology & Behavior. July 30, 2006; 88(4-5):498-505.

The amount eaten in meals by humans is a power function of the number of people present. De Castro JM, Brewer EM. Physiology & Behavior.1991; 51:121-5.

Spontaneous meal patterns of humans: influence of the presence of other people. de Castro JM, de Castro ES. American Journal of Clinical Nutrition. 1989; 50:237-47.

Impact of moods and social context on eating behavior. Patel KE, Schlundt DG. Appetite. 2001; 36:111-118.

Pleasure and alcohol: manipulating pleasantness and the acute effects of alcohol on food intake. Caton SJ, Marks JE, Hetherington MM. Physiology & Behavior. March 16, 2005; 84(3):371-7.

Dose-dependent effects of alcohol on appetite and food intake. Caton SJ, Ball M, Ahern A, Hetherinton MM. Physiology & Behavior. March 2004; 81(1):51-8.

Environmental factors that increase the food intake and consumption volume of unknowing consumers. Wansink B. Annual Review of Nutrition. 2004; 24:455-79.

Effect of ambience on food intake and food choice. Stroebele N, de Castro JM. Nutrition. September 2004; 20(9): 821-38.

Larger portion sizes lead to a sustained increase in energy intake over 2 days. Rolls BJ, Roe LS, Meengs JS. Journal of the American Dietetic Association. April 2006;106(4):543-9.

The spread of obesity in a large social network over 32 years. Christakis NA, Fowler JH. New England Journal of Medicine. July 2007;357(4):370-9.

2009 survey by Restaurants and Institutions, www.rimag.com

USDA recommendations for mercury consumption; www.usda.gov

Seafood Pocket Guide and a Sushi Pocket Guide, Environmental Defense Fund's website, www.edf.org

Chapter 6

Food cravings in a college population. Weingarten HP, Elston D. Appetite. 1991; 17: 167-175.

Meal and snack patterns are associated with dietary intake of energy and nutrirents in US adults. Kerver JM, Yang EJ, Obabyashi S, Biachi L, Song WO. Journal of the American Dietetic Association. January 2006; 106(1):46-53.

Snacking increased among U.S. adults between 1977 and 2006. Pierans C, Popkin BM. Journal of Nutrition. February 2010; 140(2):325-32.

Efficacy of eat-on-move ration for sustaining physical activity, reaction time and mood. Montain SJ, Baker-Fulco CJ, Niro PJ, Reinert AR, Cuddy JS, Ruby BC. Medicine and Science in Sports and Exercise. November 2008; 40(11):1970-6.

The role of breakfast and a mid-morning snack on the ability of children to concentrate at school. Benton D, Jarvis M. Physiology & Behavior. February 28, 2007; 90(2-3):382-5.

Drinking water is associated with weight loss in overweight dieting women independent of diet and activity. Stookey JD, Constant F, Popkin MB, Gardner CD. Obesity. November 2008; 16(11):2481-2488.

Amount of sugar consumed and recommendations re: sugar consumption, American Heart Association, and www.heart.org.

Grazing, cognitive performance and mood. Hewlett P, Smith A, Lucas E. Appetite. February 2009; 52(1):245-8.

Fasting biases brain reward systems toward high-calorie foods. Goldstone AP, de Hernandez CG, Beaver JD, Muhammed K, Croese C, Bell G, Durighel G, Hughes E, Waldman AD, Frost G, Bell JD. European Journal of Neuroscience. October 2009; 30(8): 1625-35.

Water as an essential nutrient: the physiological basis of hydration. Jequier E, Constant F. European Journal of Clinical Nutrition. February 2010; 64(2): 115-23.

Chapter 7

Statistics from the Arbitron National In-Car Study, 2009 edition; www.arbitron.com

Holiday weight management by successful weight losers and normal weight individuals. Phelan S, Wing RR, Raynor HA, Dibello J, Nedeau K, Peng W. Journal of Consulting Clinical Psychology. June 2008; 76(3):442-8.

The effect of the Thanksgiving holiday on weight gain. Hull HR, Radley D, Dinger MK, Fields DA. Nutrition Journal. November 21, 2006; 5:29.

A prospective study of holiday weight gain. Yanovski JA, Yanovski SZ, Sovik KN, Nguyen TT, O'Neil PM, Sebring NG. New England Journal of Medicine March 23, 2000; 342(12):861-7.

Short-term appetite control in response to a 6-week exercise programme in sedentary volunteers. Martins C, Truby H, Morgan LM. British Journal of Nutrition. October 2007; 98(4):834-42.

The effect of an incremental increase in exercise on appetite, eating behavior and energy balance in lean men and women feeding ad libitum. Whybrow S, Hughes DA, Ritz P, Johnstone AM, Horgan GW, King N, Blundell JE, Stubbs RJ. British Journal of Nutrition. November 2008; 100(5):1109-15.

Sleep curtailment is accompanied by increased intake of calories from snacks. Nedeltcheva AV, Kilkus JM, Imperial J, Kasza K, Schoeller DA, Penev PD. American Journal of Clinical Nutrition. January 2009; 89(1):126-33.

Acute partial sleep deprivation increases food intake in healthy men. Brondel L, Romer MA, Nougues PM, Touyarou P, Davenne D. American Journal of Clinical Nutrition. June 2010; 91(6):1550-9.

Chapter 8

2008 Stress in America poll, American Psychology Association, www.apa.org

Relationship between stress, eating behavior, and obesity. Torres SJ, Nowson CA. Nutrition. November-December 2007;23(11-12):887-94.

Common risk factors for changes in body weight and psychological well-being in Japanese male middle-aged workers. Sagara T, Hitomi Y, Kambayashi Y, Hibino Y, Matsuzaki I, Sasahara S, Ogino K, Hatta K, Nkamura H. Environmental Health and Preventive Medicine. November 2009;14(6):329-27.

Psychological stress and change in weight among US adults. Block JP, He Y, Zaslavsky AM, Ding L, Ayanian JZ. American Journal of Epidemiology. July 15, 2009;170(2):181-92.

Soothing music can increase oxytocin levels during bed rest after open-heart surgery: a randomised control trial. Nilsson U. Journal of Clinical Nursing. August 2009;18(15):2153-61.

Healing the wounds of organizational injustice: examining the benefits of expressive writing. Barclay LJ, Skarlicki DP. Journal of Applied Psychology. March 2009;94(2):511-23.

Effects of physical activity intensity, frequency, and activity type on 10-y weight change in middle-aged men and women. Littman AJ, Kristal AR, White E. International Journal of Obesity. May 2005;29(5):524-33.

Fifteen-year longitudinal trends in walking patterns and their impact on weight change. Gordon-Larsen P, Hou N, Sidney S, Sternfield B, Lewis CE, Jacobs DR Jr, Popkin BM. American Journal of Clinical Nutrition. January 2009;89(1):19-26.

Relations of exercise, self-appraisal, mood changes and weight loss in obese women: testing propositions based on Baker and Brownell's (2000) model. Annesi JJ, Unruh JL. American Journal of Medicine and Science. March 2008;335(3):198-204.

10,000 steps a day recommendation, http://www.shapeup.org/shape/steps.php

Effect of music on perceived exertion, plasma lactate, norepinephrine and cardiovascular hemodynamics during treadmill running. Szmedra L, Bacharach DW. International Journal of Sports Medicine. January 1998;19(1):32-7.

The association between sleep duration and weight gain in adults: a 6-year prospective study from the Quebec Family Study. Chaput JP, Després JP, Bouchard C, Tremblay. Sleep. April 1, 2008;31(4):517-23.

The effects of a poor night sleep on mood, cognitive, autonomic and electrophysiological measures. Barnett KJ, Cooper NJ. Journal of Integrated Neuroscience. September 2008;7(3):405-20.

Poor reported sleep quality predicts low positive effect in daily life among healthy and mood-disordered persons. Bower B, Bylsma LM, Morris BH, Rottenberg J. Journal of Sleep Research. March 31, 2010; 2010 Mar 31. [epub ahead of print]

Insomnia with objective short sleep duration is associated with deficits in neuropsychological performance: a general population study. Fernandez-Mendoza J, Calhoun S, Bixler EO, Pejovic S, Karataraki M, Liao D, Vela-Bueno A, Ramos-Platon MJ, Sauder KA, Vgontzas AN. Sleep. April 1, 2010;33(4):459-65.

Sleep statistics, National Sleep Foundation, www. nationalsleepfoundation.org

Very happy people. Diener E, Seligman ME. Psychological Science. January 2002:13(1):81-4.

Women's perceived body image: relations with personal happiness. Stokes R, Frederick-Recascino C. Journal of Women and Aging. 2003; 15(1):17029.

Effect of forced laughter on mood. Foley E, Matheis R, Schaefer C. Psychological Reports. February 2002;90(1):184.

Spending money on others promotes happiness. Dunn EW, Aknin LB, Norton MI. Science. March 21, 2008; 319(5870):1687-8.

Is happiness having what you want, wanting what you have, or both? Larsen JT, McKibban AR. Psychological Science. April 2008;19(4):371-7.

The association between exercise participation and well-being: a co-twin study. Stubbe JH, de Moor MH, Boomsma DI, de Geus EJ. Preventive Medicine. February 2007; 44(2):148-52.

Doing well by doing good. The relationship between formal volunteering and self-reported health and happiness. Borgonovi F. Social Science & Medicine. June 2008; 66(11):2321-34.

2008 Australian Happiness Index, http://www.seductionlabs. org/2008/10/02/what-makes-men-and-women-happy/

Sexual well-being, happiness and satisfaction, in women: the case for a new conceptual paradigm. Rosen RC, Bachmann GA. Journal of Sexuality and Marital Therapy.2008;34(4):291-7.

INDEX

Available from NorlightsPress and fine booksellers everywhere

Toll free: 888-558-4354   **Online:** www.norlightspress.com
Shipping Info: Add $2.95 for first item and $1.00 for each additional item

Name _____

Address _____

Daytime Phone _____

E-mail _____

No. Copies	Title	Price (each)	Total Cost

	Subtotal	
	Shipping	
	Total	

Payment by (circle one):

   Check   Visa   Mastercard   Discover   Am Express

Card number_____3 digit code_____

Exp.date_____ Signature_____

Mailing Address:
2721 Tulip Tree Rd.
Nashville, IN 47448

Sign up to receive our catalogue at www.norlightspress.com

LaVergne, TN USA
15 October 2010
200962LV00003B/1/P